Run for Health...

The aim of the CONSUMER GUIDE® Running Program is simple: to condition your heart and lungs and strengthen them through the most effective exercise for that purpose — running.

Run for Serenity...

In this workaday world, so filled with hassles, tension and unrest, the glorious release found by runners is one of the best natural tranquilizers.

Run for Fun...

Most of us already have enough pressure in our lives. Running ought to take some of the pressure off. If you want to run, you want to enjoy your running.

Run for Energy...

Working capacity is, of course, linked to endurance and stamina. With conditioning comes a greater capacity to get things done. You are able to do more before feeling fatigued. In short, you have more pep.

Run for Insight...

Most runners start out with the simple aim of toning up their bodies and expanding their oxygen supply. But they often stick to it when they find they are expanding their consciousness as well. They like what running is doing for their thinking.

Run for Exhilaration...

The CONSUMER GUIDE® Running Program does not ask more of you than you can reasonably do. We want to get you started, keep you going, and help you finally experience the physical, mental, and emotional exhilaration that comes from running with ease.

BY THE EDITORS OF CONSUMER GUIDE®

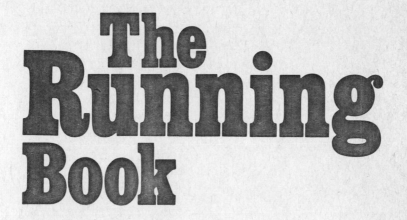

The Running Book

Beekman House
New York

Library of Congress Catalog Card Number: 78-58613

This edition published by:
Beekman House
A Division of Crown Publishers, Inc.
One Park Avenue
New York, N.Y. 10016
By arrangement with Publications International, Ltd.

Cover Photo: Converse Rubber Company
Illustrator: Steven Boswick

Contents

Contents

Contents

Introduction

WHY IS everyone so excited about running? What makes so many thousands of amateur athletes compete in grueling marathons? What motivates all those people jogging down the streets at dawn? Is running really all it's cracked up to be — or is it just another fad, doomed to oblivion like hula hoops and coonskin caps?

We believe that running is here to stay. There's something special about knowing your body is doing what it's meant to do. In this workaday world, so filled with hassles, tension, and un-

Introduction

rest, the glorious release found by runners is one of the best natural tranquilizers. The runner leaves care and worry behind and communes with nature and with his or her own body. Just ask any runner.

Running, also known as jogging (the two terms are generally used interchangeably), is one of the most pleasurable sports you can participate in. It's also one of the healthiest. Unlike most popular games and sports, running is terrific exercise. While you're enjoying the fresh air and a sense of accomplishment, your heart and lungs are receiving a great workout. Sustained cardiovascular exertion is the key to physical fitness, and running is one of the most — if not *the* most — effective ways of achieving it.

Perhaps you are among the millions who have been thinking about running, inspired by all the enthusiasts you see and all the benefits you read about. Perhaps you have even investigated many of the running programs now available, only to be discouraged by the formidable requirements they set up. *The Running Book* is for you.

The unique CONSUMER GUIDE® running program is designed to transform the chair-bound wistful thinker into an active and energetic doer as painlessly as possible. Developed by Charles Kuntzleman, the national consultant on physical fitness to the YMCA, this program allows you to progress at your own rate. You compete only with yourself, and not against any arbitrary standards that may be beyond your abilities. You move ahead as quickly or as slowly as you like, reaping all the wonderful benefits of running from the very beginning.

The Running Book contains all the information you need to get the most out of your program. Running shoes? You'll find an entire chapter devoted to these essential pieces of equipment — including brand-name evaluations and recommendations. You'll also learn how to prevent and cope with injuries, what to do when you can't run, and where to go for more information.

Who ran the very first marathon? What's the world record for 1500 meters? Do you have Morton's toe? Why is a stress test important? Are "Fun Runs" really fun?

The Running Book answers all these questions — and many more. Join the millions of happy joggers who have discovered the marvelous world of running!

What Running Will Do For You

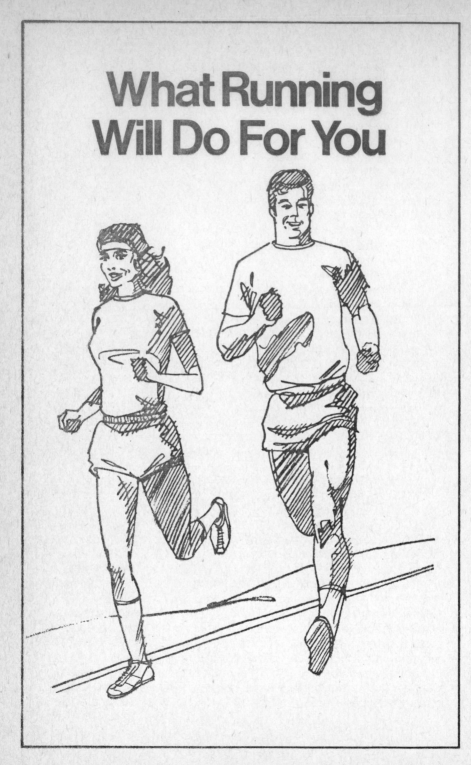

Benefits Of Running

IF YOU want to learn what motivates runners and get a good idea of just what running can do for you, you might go out, as we did, and stop a number of people jogging through neighborhoods or city parks and ask. We put it as simply as we could: "Why do you do it day after day?"

"Because my doctor said I'd better do *something* or I'd end up with a heart attack."

"I sat on my duff all day and never got any exercise."

"I was really bored."

"No energy. I was pooped all the time, for no reason."

"It's fun!"

"I was drinking too much."

You get the idea. Show us a roomful of runners and we'll show you a roomful of reasons.

We'll also show you a cross-section of life: the elderly; the middle-aged; the young; the healthy and the not-so-healthy; vigorous athletic types and those who once felt like Robert Hutchins, the former President of the University of Chicago. Whenever he was tempted to indulge in a little exercise, he said, he promptly laid down until the inclination passed.

Join The Primitives

Two million years ago a world full of runners wasn't an extraordinary thing. Running was the best way to get around, find food, escape from one's enemies, and welcome one's friends. Today, some Australian aborigines still run to secure the basic necessities of life. They chase a kangaroo mile after mile for days — running, walking, then running again until the kangaroo is too exhausted to go any farther. Then they kill it for food and carry their catch back the way they came — running and walking, mile after mile, until they arrive again at their home camp.

That's what you call endurance. There are a few other peoples scattered through the mountain regions of Pakistan, Ecuador, and the U.S.S.R. who have that kind of stamina and

Benefits Of Running

lead similar lives. They use their bodies vigorously every day, in everything they do. It's a simpler life than the one we are accustomed to, but one that is much more physically active than that of people working in our technological society. They live out an existence we call "primitive," but, for the most part, they live 20 or 30 years longer than the average sedentary worker in more "advanced" societies where machinery is certainly labor-saving, but hardly life-saving. Many of these "primitive" peoples reach ages of 100 years and more, vigorous to the end.

Today's runners are, in a way, 20th-Century primitives of this sort. They've come to see the simple logic of the body, what makes it work and what makes it wither. So they've gotten out of their cars and up from their easy chairs and away from their TV sets and off the bar stools and begun to connect with sidewalks and roads, grasslands and paths, wind, sunshine, and rain. As Dr. George Sheehan, heart specialist, runner, and prominent writer on running says: "For every runner who tours the world running marathons, there are thousands who run to hear the leaves and listen to rain and look to the day when it is all suddenly as easy as a bird in flight."

These are the people who practice the long, slow, distance runs. They run because running gives them sheer pleasure, and they declare almost universally that after they have been going for about 45 minutes to an hour they experience an extraordinary feeling of euphoria. Filled with energy, they are literally "high" on running.

It's a matter of balance, a psychological high, the body and mind working together in a kind of ideal unity. We're all familiar with the way psychosomatic disease works. The body and mind, inseparably bound together, pull a person into a downward spiral of disorder. There's no reason to think the high we're describing is any different. The body is doing what it does best and helping the mind to do what it does best. The well-being of one nourishes the well-being of the other and the "thrust" of the experience is "upward." The "high" is simply the peak of that thrust, produced by the harmonious balance between body and mind.

More and more, physical fitness experts and physicians are coming to the conclusion that running is one of the best ways to achieve that balance. They are beginning to act on what they probably have known all along — that a sense of well-being can to a great extent depend on the physiological machine we call the human body.

Your
Amazing Body

It's the most complicated machine of all and it needs a lot of things to keep it going, oxygen above all. You can deprive yourself of food for weeks, or water for days. But just try holding your breath for more than a few minutes and see what happens. Oxygen is vital if you want to stay alive. It must pass through the lungs and into every cell of that complicated machine. And it all depends on a simple pump. But what a pump! Your heart is an incredibly efficient organ, and does its job night and day with no more rest than the split second between beats. The human heart usually beats between 60 and 80 times a minute. In the average person, the heart beats about 70 to 72 times each minute, or a little over one beat per second. At each beat, even under the most restful conditions, the heart pumps about 130 cubic centimeters of blood so that it pumps five liters (a little over five quarts) of blood each minute. To give you a better idea of how hard your heart works to keep you alive, if you should be lucky enough to live to 100, your heart will beat some four billion times. The work done by your heart during that long period is the equivalent of lifting 70 pounds off the ground every minute of your life.

Your heart does deserve a little consideration in return. There are a number of physical activities that have come to be known as "aerobic exercises" which promote the health of the heart while increasing the body's ability to utilize oxygen. Swimming, rowing, walking, cycling — any exercise or sport, in

Benefits Of Running

fact, that requires sustained activity over a long period — are aerobic exercises. But running heads the list. Dr. Kenneth Cooper, who developed the concept of aerobics and was perhaps the person most responsible for bringing it to wide public attention, has this to say about the relative merit of running as an aerobic exercise: "If you were to ask me . . . what exercise can be used most effectively, I'd have no hesitancy about recommending running. As one of my runners put it, 'It's like a dry martini. You get more for your money — and quicker.' "

The "more" you get for your money can range from controlling your weight to saving your life. Countless studies show that while the heart of the average sedentary person beats about 70 times each minute at rest, the heart of a long-distance runner generally beats only 30 to 35 times each minute. While beating at half the average rate, it circulates oxygen-rich blood throughout the body, sending oxygen to the cells. How can this happen when the heart is only working at half-power?

The truth is that the heart conditioned by long-distance running beats more strongly and deeply. Since the lungs of the long-distance runner also become highly conditioned, the heart and lungs working together take in more oxygen during a given time and distribute it more efficiently throughout the body. The conditioned runner's heart, working at half the average rate, gets more rest between beats and will last longer. That 100-year-old heart we mentioned earlier would have beat only two billion times instead of four billion.

Besides having stronger hearts, well-conditioned runners tend to have slender bodies. Dr. Peter Wood, a biochemist at Stanford University, reports that a research study he did of runners between the ages of 35 and 65 disclosed that many had the physical conditioning of people half their ages. They had extraordinary endurance and were as lean as most 20-year-olds.

But running is not the whole story behind that kind of weight control. Losing weight and maintaining your new weight at the appropriate level depends on the proper balance between your intake of calories and your expenditure of energy. In short, between how much you eat and how much you move around. Any calories not used up in activity such as walking, running,

Benefits Of Running

scrubbing floors, playing racquetball, cycling, typing a letter, or combing your hair are stored in the body as fat. It's that simple. So the less active you are, the more likely you are to put on pounds. If you are overweight, merely running will not solve the problem. It will help, though, because every step you run will burn up calories.

To solve an overweight problem you'll have to pay a little more attention to what you put on your plate every day and how often you go through this necessary ritual. Your particular ritual may turn out to be less difficult to change than you expect. Many new joggers report changes in their patterns of eating and drinking as they begin to get into the swing of the sport. In fact, most runners say that a desire to eat differently appeared once they started a program of regular running. One person we talked to, for example, found that he was eating more fish and chicken and less meat than he did before he became a runner. With less meat in his diet, he took in fewer fattening calories.

If you're luckier than most and don't have to keep letting out your belt another notch, don't worry about becoming a walking bag of bones if you take up running several times a week. Your body knows how to regulate itself, so the chances are that you will start taking in more calories to meet the new demands of your body for more energy. You may even gain a pound or two after you start to run, but this probably will take the form of muscle rather than fat.

Many women find that jogging helps to trim their hips and thighs, troublesome areas that, like the male paunch, seem to strike fat cells as attractive places to colonize. Jogging can chase these fat cells away, but they'll be right back when you stop the exercise. Sporadic exercise is like fad dieting — any benefits you receive are only temporary. There are, however, conditions much more serious than a paunch or secretary's spread. For example, heart disease. Every year about 700,000 Americans die because their hearts stop pumping. Heart specialists used to advise their cardiac patients to, "Take it easy. Rest a lot. Don't overwork yourself." Some doctors still give that advice. More and more, however, the benefits of vigorous walking, jogging, running, or a combination of these are being recognized as the best way to avoid disability and premature death from heart conditions.

Running For Heart And Head

Dr. Cooper confidently says that "the days of the 'take it easy' cures are long gone" and is glad of it. "They only compound the problem," he adds. Cooper and others who conduct exercise rehabilitation programs for cardiac patients have extensive experience with the beneficial effects of running on diseases of the heart. One of his "Poopers," as he calls them, had a congenital heart defect that required surgery. "The surgery was successful but he couldn't regain his strength. We started training him and before long he was running a mile in 7½ minutes and a mile and a half in 12½ minutes. Not bad for a man following open-heart surgery. . . . He tried 'taking it easy' after his operation and got worse. He began exercising and got better."

The Cleveland YMCA conducts a rehabilitation program for patients who have had heart attacks. The program begins gradually and works up to a full hour of calisthenics, 15 minutes of walking/running, and recreational volleyball. Dr. Herman Hellerstein of Cleveland, who examined one group, reported that the resting heart rate in some had dropped as much as 20 beats per minute. In addition, their cholesterol and triglyceride (fat) levels had fallen and circulation had improved.

"An ounce of prevention is worth a pound of cure," goes the maxim. The examples we've cited show quite clearly that starting to run *after* a heart attack can bring life-saving benefits, but anyone with an ounce of sense would be wise to start getting into condition *before* a heart attack strikes.

Cooper, Hellerstein, and the Cleveland YMCA are interested primarily in what running can do for the body, especially the heart. Dr. Thaddeus Kostrubala, a psychiatrist, is mainly interested in what running can do for people's heads. But it was his heart that first brought him to discover the benefits of running. A physician told him to either lose weight and get himself

Benefits Of Running

into decent physical condition or to expect his heart to stop pumping. Now he uses running as one mode of therapy for his psychiatric patients. In an experiment with one group, he ran with them for one hour, three times a week, after which he conducted group sessions. During these sessions the patients were encouraged to express the thoughts and feelings that surfaced during their runs.

In the course of time nearly all members of the group reported major changes taking place in their behavior and attitudes. Many were smoking and drinking less than before. Depressions were lifting. Unhealthy relationships were either being straightened out or broken off. A woman who had lost interest in eating and weighed only 79 pounds regained her appetite for food during her running therapy. Over a period of 18 months she gained more than 50 pounds. Another person, a heroin addict, actually freed himself of his habit, and replaced his drug "high" with the runner's "high" so often compared to that drug experience. A patient who was considered an incurable paranoid schizophrenic recovered to such an extent that he now maintains a B average in college and has a steady job. Today he uses no medication and lives without any identifiable trace of his former disease.

We do not guarantee any direct connection between running and the cure of mental and emotional disease. If you suffer from problems of this nature, don't go jogging and expect them to disappear. Instead, see a doctor. We present these examples merely to show one physician's practical recognition of the intimate relationship that exists between body and mind.

Most of us, happily, simply suffer from the ordinary psychological blahs, the garden-variety tensions and stress common in modern life. Running can help you get rid of them.

You can also expect a corresponding "tune-up" to take place in your mind. Not necessarily the "high" we mentioned above, but something quite close to it. Most runners start out with the simple aim of toning up their bodies and expanding their oxygen supply. But they often stick to it when they find that they are expanding their consciousness as well. They like what running is doing for their thinking.

For one thing, it sweeps away a lot of the mental cobwebs that have been hanging around inside the head for so long.

Benefits Of Running

Most runners say they begin to feel their capacities picking up in all areas of their lives as they begin to feel better physically. This does not mean that you will be transformed into a genius simply by running a few miles a week. But if you are reasonably competent in your work, it is very possible that running will open up some blocked doorways to imaginative thinking and enable you to make better use of what you know. As Joe Henderson, editor of *Runner's World* puts it, "Running won't turn an Edith Bunker into a Barbara Walters." But — if you can imagine Edith Bunker in running shoes — running can make it possible for Edith to be a much more interesting Edith.

One author we talked with, for example, said that there is a practical connection between running and writing, in her case at least. Running clears her mind for writing. Her ideas seem to flow more easily from her mind to the page. So she gets up early every morning and runs for an hour before facing the typewriter. One businessman we know jogs for 30 minutes at lunch every working day and claims that he works far more productively in the afternoons than he ever did before.

Other runners have testified to similar benefits. One young professional told us that running changed the direction of his life. To reach his present position in his corporation he had habitually worked 14- and 15-hour days. He wanted to succeed and, to his mind, the way to succeed was to take on more and more responsibility, get to work earlier, and leave later. That didn't leave much time for anything but work. Finally his wife got fed up with it, packed up the kids, and left. That was enough to make him question his whole outlook. "Something's got to change," he thought, and decided it was himself. He took a little bit of those 15-hour days and started running. He's still running. Now he has chucked the 15-hour routine altogether. He finds he can get the same work done in not much more than the eight hours of a normal workday. And although no one claims that running is a panacea for all marital woes, in this particular case his wife came back and now they jog together.

Those of you who can commit yourselves to running daily, or at least several times a week, and keep at it will eventually reap the physical benefits we've been talking about, we promise you. The other benefits, we don't promise. But we won't be surprised if they fall into your lap. We hope they do.

Don't Get Discouraged

In any case, prepare yourself for one difficult part — the early pain of doing something you're not used to doing. Jack Batten, who started exercising seriously at the age of 44, kept a diary of each day's workout. Mostly he ran. On the first day he felt mild pains, especially in his joints. He remained undisturbed and optimistic about his new venture. The second day he awoke to ticks, twinges, spasms, and assorted muscular agonies running through his body, especially in his legs. But he persevered. By day 10 he was disillusioned. Would the pain never end? Why, in heaven's name, was he going through all this? By the 25th day he had to force himself to head for the gym. His fitness counselor told him to "hang in there."

He did. And by the 55th day of his program things were different. The aches and the pains were mostly gone, but not the memory of that early suffering.

His case was extreme and probably caused by overenthusiasm. Perhaps a better word would be indiscretion. It doesn't have to be all that painful. Those early days of running do require toil and persistence, but not punishment.

The program we recommend to you later in the book is free of punishment, but not of work. For any fitness program to be effective it has to be pursued week after week, month after month. It has to suit your temperament and your body and become part of the way you live.

We think that a running program designed for the majority of people should be flexible enough to make that happen. We have seen too many exercisers and potential runners disillusioned by awesome programs that ended with the individual back in front of his TV set drinking beer with his running shoes in the closet gathering dust.

Most of us already have enough pressure in our lives. Running ought to take some of the pressure off. If you want to run, you want to enjoy your running, not be hounded by it. That is

Benefits Of Running

why you are the most appropriate person to set your running course and your running goals.

So, before you set out on a lope around the block, take a good look at yourself. How old are you? If you are 40 or 65 your approach to jogging will have to be a little different from the way an 18-year old would go about it. How fit are you? If you are already in fairly good shape, then you can expect to advance through the stages of the running program more quickly.

If you have any health problems now — asthma perhaps or a heart condition — you will need to take that into account while working through your program. Elsewhere in this book we emphasize the absolute necessity of having a medical check-up before you begin any program of running. Obviously, that precaution is doubly necessary in your case.

Whether you are a man or a woman, a child or a senior citizen, healthy as a horse or plagued by ailments, running can help you. "At your own pace." Those are the words to remember. The beautiful thing is that running is a very individual endeavor. Look at yourself. Decide what *you* want from running. And go after *that*.

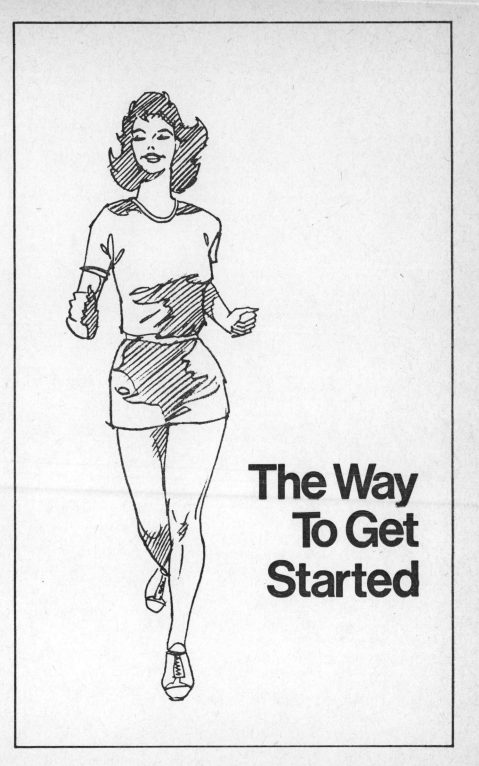

The Way To Get Started

Getting Started

IF YOU now feel an overwhelming urge to jump into a pair of running shoes, rush out the door, and surprise your neighbors with your new-found enthusiasm for exercise — don't. We certainly want you to run. And we want you to share the joy that is a part of vigorous exercise. But, above all, we want you to go about it in the right way — for the sake of the pleasure and for the sake of your health. Be enthusiastic but be sensible.

We said before that running is for everyone. Anybody can do it — men, women, the young, the elderly, the healthy, and the ailing. The body was made for running. Despite all the ballyhoo from the fashion industry about clothes designed for running, to run costs nothing, or almost nothing: a pair of running shoes, if you want to spare your feet. That's about all.

Once you've started, who knows? You'll probably become one of a great number for whom running is as natural a habit as brushing teeth.

See Your Doctor First

But before you start, it is very important that you *check with your doctor*. Running should contribute to your health in very general and specific ways. You must be certain that it cannot harm you in any way.

Although running experts may disagree on training methods, running techniques, or other details touching on the sport, all of them strongly advocate one thing: anyone about to undertake a program of any sustained, vigorous exercise such as running should have a thorough medical check-up beforehand. We subscribe completely to this important precaution. See your physician, tell him what you plan to do, have him examine you, ask for his advice, and then follow it.

It is true that under doctor's orders some victims of heart attacks have turned to running as therapy and have improved their condition so much that they might conceivably be able to finish the grueling Boston Marathon. Many others, while not up

Getting Started

to competing in a marathon, nonetheless have become very accomplished runners with hearts stronger than they've been in years. But not all heart attack victims or potential victims should embark on a running program. Some diseases and ailments — such as advanced arthritis, diabetes, consistent pains in the lower back, orthopedic problems, and various conditions of the liver and kidneys — make sustained running impossible. If you know that you have one of these conditions and still want to work on a regular program of exercise to improve your overall fitness, your doctor should be able to suggest one that suits your physical limitations.

Even if you feel confident that you don't have any of these ailments, you still would be well advised to have a medical examination. You may have one of these diseases without yet knowing it. Some other medical factor may also rule running out for you. Sure, you never felt better in your life, you're healthy as a horse, fit as a fiddle, and so on. But after all, the main reason you want to take this step in the first place is to improve your general well-being. And if you're not as healthy as you think you are, you might end up with results you hadn't bargained for.

Once in the doctor's office, make certain he includes an electrocardiogram (ECG) in the examination. If you tell him you plan to run, it isn't likely he will omit this. It is one of the most important tests he can give you. It evaluates the performance of the heart and reveals any abnormalities that might force you to abandon the idea altogether or at least modify your running program.

Two kinds of ECG examinations are generally available to test the heart: the normal ECG and the stress ECG, usually called a *stress test*. The normal ECG tests your heart while you are lying down. Consequently, it does not show how your heart performs when it is working under stress, as it will be while running.

The stress test, on the other hand, essentially duplicates the conditions of running as closely as possible by means of a treadmill. You walk, then run on the treadmill at progressively faster speeds and at steeper angles. This steadily increases the stress your heart is under and causes it to beat faster and faster. Electronic devices record your heart rate and monitor the heart's key functions until your exertion raises your heart beat to about 75% of your maximum rate. (Maximum heart rate and the method for determining it for yourself are discussed in detail in "A Running Program Designed For You.") Not many doctors are equipped to conduct a stress test in their offices, but they will send you to a clinic or hospital which has the necessary facilities for running the test.

It should be noted that a stress ECG is not inexpensive. They usually run slightly over $100. That may cool you toward them, but they are worthwhile if you can afford one. In any case, an ordinary medical check-up that includes a normal ECG is essential, regardless of the cost.

Fitness Tests

Several fitness tests have been devised that you can perform yourself, but they should not replace the medical check-up. These tests are primarily useful in giving you a rough idea of your conditioning at the beginning of, and during, your running program. We warn you that these tests are strenuous and should be attempted only with caution if you have not already been exercising on a regular basis. In fact, we recommend that you try these tests *after* receiving your doctor's okay.

The Step Test

This test has a number of variations and goes by several names. In *The Complete Book of Running,* James Fixx calls it the Harvard Step Test, while the *Official YMCA Physical Fitness Handbook* refers to it as the Kasch Pulse Recovery Test. In both versions of the test you perform an exercise that raises your heartbeat to a certain level, depending on your condition. Then you compare that rate to a given standard to determine your relative degree of fitness. You step up onto a bench with one foot, then with the other; return the first foot to the floor, then the other, to complete the cycle. Perform this complete cycle of step-up, step-down 30 times a minute for four minutes. The height of the bench depends upon your height.

One minute after you stop, take your pulse for 30 seconds

Getting Started

The Step Test

It is important to use a bench of the proper height if you want an accurate assessment of your condition. Obviously, a short person would expend a great deal more energy mounting and dismounting than a tall person if they used benches of the same height.

If You Are	The Bench Should Be
Under 5' tall	12" high
5' 1" to 5' 3" tall	14" high
5' 3" to 5' 9" tall	16" high
5' 9" to 6' tall	18" high
Over 6' tall	20" high

and record the number of pulses you feel during that period. Repeat this at two minutes and three minutes (counting for 30 seconds each time) after the completion of the exercise. Add up the three 30-second pulse counts and multiply the sum by two. Divide the result into the total time spent exercising multiplied by 100.

For example, if your pulse rate was 50 after one minute, 45 after two minutes, and 40 after three minutes, you would:
Add the three counts:
$$50 + 45 + 40 = 135$$
Multiply by two to convert the 30-second counts into 60-second counts:
$$135 \times 2 = 270$$
Multiply the number of seconds you exercised by 100:
240 seconds (4 minutes) $\times$ 100 = 24,000
Divide your pulse rate into the time:
$$24,000 \div 270 = 88.8$$
Then compare the result with the following scale:

Score	Rating
Above 90	Excellent
81 to 90	Very Good
71 to 80	Good
61 to 70	Fair
Below 60	Poor

Getting Started

If you are unable to continue the test for the full four minutes, you can forget the math. Just put yourself in the "Poor" category. Don't be discouraged, however. Most people will start out in this category and a fitness program will improve your condition surprisingly soon.

The Kasch Test

The Kasch test is a little different and mathematically a lot simpler. Do the same exercise, but with only 24 step-ups and step-downs per minute for a period of three minutes. Five seconds after you stop, take your pulse rate for one minute and compare it to this chart:

Pulse Rate	Rating
75 to 79	Excellent
80 to 94	Good
95 to 119	Average
120 to 129	Fair
130 and above	Poor

The Cooper Test

This test is part of Dr. Cooper's scientific, goal-oriented, and relatively demanding fitness program. It ascertains your relative fitness according to the distance you are able to cover in 12 minutes of running, walking, or crawling — any way you can manage to make it. You will need a pre-measured track for a testing ground. The most common ones are usually a quarter-mile long. If you can't find a convenient track, you can measure a route with your automobile. When your 12 minutes are up, calculate the distance you have covered and compare it to Dr. Cooper's chart.

The Balke Test

This test, originated by an authority on physiology, determines the body's relative fitness by measuring its capacity to utilize oxygen, that is, its maximum oxygen uptake, when engaged in sustained exercise. The higher the uptake, the greater the fit-

The 12-Minute Running/Walking Test*

This demanding test measures the distance you are able to cover in 12 minutes. You may run or walk, depending on your condition and abilities. *Do not attempt this test without your doctor's permission unless you limit yourself to walking.*

Fitness	Age Group (years)					
	13 to 19	20 to 29	30 to 39	40 to 49	50 to 59	60+
Distance In Miles For Men						
Superior	1.87+	1.77+	1.70+	1.66+	1.59+	1.56+
Excellent	1.73-1.86	1.65-1.76	1.57-1.69	1.54-1.65	1.45-1.58	1.33-1.55
Good	1.57-1.72	1.50-1.64	1.46-1.56	1.40-1.53	1.31-1.44	1.21-1.32
Fair	1.38-1.56	1.32-1.49	1.31-1.45	1.25-1.39	1.17-1.30	1.03-1.20
Poor	1.30-1.37	1.22-1.31	1.18-1.30	1.14-1.24	1.03-1.16	0.87-1.02
Very poor	Under 1.30	Uncer 1.22	Under 1.18	Under 1.14	Under 1.03	Under 0.87
Distance In Miles For Women						
Superior	1.52+	1.46+	1.40+	1.35+	1.31+	1.19+
Excellent	1.44-1.51	1.35-1.45	1.30-1.39	1.25-1.34	1.19-1.30	1.10-1.18
Good	1.30-1.43	1.23-1.34	1.19-1.29	1.12-1.24	1.06-1.18	0.99-1.09
Fair	1.19-1.29	1.12-1.22	1.06-1.18	0.99-1.11	0.94-1.05	0.87-0.98
Poor	1.00-1.18	0.96-1.11	0.95-1.05	0.88-0.98	0.84-0.93	0.78-0.86
Very poor	Under 1.00	Under 0.96	Under 0.94	Under 0.88	Under 0.84	Under 0.78

*Charts based on those of Kenneth Cooper in *The Aerobics Way* (New York, M. Evans, 1977).

Maximum Oxygen Uptake

The amount of oxygen used by your body during sustained exercise is an excellent way of measuring your fitness. Calculate your oxygen uptake as explained in the text and compare your result with the chart.*

Fitness Rating

	Age Group				
	20 to 29	30 to 39	40 to 49	50 to 59	60+
			For Men		
Excellent	54+	50+	46+	44+	40+
Good	53 to 45	49 to 43	45 to 40	43 to 38	39 to 35
Average	44 to 40	42 to 35	39 to 33	37 to 31	34 to 29
Fair	39 to 33	34 to 27	32 to 25	30 to 22	28 to 21
Poor	Under 33	Under 27	Under 25	Under 22	Under 21
			For Women		
Excellent	50+	46+	42+	38+	—
Good	48 to 44	45 to 41	41 to 37	37 to 32	—
Average	43 to 35	40 to 34	36 to 30	32 to 27	—
Fair	34 to 29	33 to 28	29 to 24	26 to 21	—
Poor	Under 29	Under 28	Under 24	Under 21	—

*Adapted from Jack Batten, *The Complete Jogger* (New York, Harcourt Brace Jovanovich, 1977).

Getting Started

ness. In this test you are asked to walk, jog, run, etc., for 15 minutes. The distance you cover in that time is then measured in *meters* (1609.354 meters to one mile). The distance covered is divided by 15. This will give you your speed in meters per minute. Now, to figure your maximum oxygen uptake, you make the following calculations:

Your speed minus 133 times .172 plus 33.3

For example, if you covered exactly two miles in 15 minutes, you would:

Multiply 1609.354 by two to find your speed in meters:

1609.354 × 2 = 3218.708

Divide by 15 to find your speed in meters per minute:

3218.708 ÷ 15 = 214.6

Subtract 133:

214.6 − 133 = 81.6

Multiply by .172:

81.6 × .172 = 14.03

Add 33.3:

14.03 + 33.3 = 47.33

It all may look a bit complicated, but the result you end up with represents the amount of oxygen your body can process at a given rate. And that, in a nutshell, is what running is all about. To find out where your maximum oxygen uptake would place you on a scale of relative fitness, compare the result of your calculations to the chart.

Let Your Body Talk To You

These tests may be useful for some people, but not for others. If mathematics and formulas are not your cup of tea, there is a very simple way for you to get a rough idea of how fit you are — both before you begin to run and during your running program. Just let your body talk to you. Start out with a walk or an easy

Getting Started

jog. Feel what happens. Are you breathing heavily after only two blocks of brisk walking? Or can you go on for miles? Does a gentle jog have you puffing after the first dozen or so yards? Your body reacts to stress automatically and wastes no time in letting you know how it feels. So pay attention to it. And don't try to make it do more work than it can before it builds up a little stamina.

It takes time to build stamina. And it takes pretty rigorous exercise. An unexercised body needs a period of pre-conditioning before it gets into real training. Most running programs begin with pre-conditioning exercises. One of the best of these is simple walking. In fact, you can begin your own pre-conditioning activity even before you actually start on your program, or even before you see your doctor. Just start walking. Leave your wheels behind if the trip is not too far. Walk to the hardware store on Saturday morning, walk to the movies, visit your friends with your feet instead of your car. Try to break the habit of reaching for your car keys. Stifle the urge to drive every place you have to go. The sidewalks won't wear out. Use them.

If it's convenient, walk to work. It not, park your car farther from the office or train station than is your habit and walk the rest of the way. Stay away from elevators and escalators. Use the stairs. If your office is located too many floors up in the building for this, take the stairs part of the way and make the rest of the trip in the elevator. Make a brisk after-dinner walk for 10 or 15 minutes a regular part of your evening. Very likely, if you get into habits like these, it won't be long before you feel the urge to run, and to run on a regular basis.

When you do get into running itself, the point is not to win races, but to build up your endurance. Joe Henderson, editor of *Runner's World* and a runner for 20 years, suggests that the beginning runner should "aim low, work easy, sacrifice nothing." Roy Ald, physical fitness instructor and author of *Jogging, Aerobics and Diet,* uses a simple word to remind his students of the importance of going slowly at first: *EASE,* he says, is the key word in a running program. *E,* for endurance, the key to aerobic fitness, the thing you are trying to build through long, slow, distance running; *A,* for agility, the quick, active movement you have when your muscles and joints are working together smoothly; *S,* for the strength which your body begins to possess, making you less susceptible to infections; *E,* for the energy a body is filled with when oxygen flows easily to all its parts. Ease into a program of running. That's the right approach.

A Special Word To Women

If you are a woman, we want to suggest some special precautions for you as you prepare to run. Your heart and lung capacities are lower than those of a man, so you do not need to jog or run as hard as he does to reach the same level of fitness. This is so because, for the same degree of exertion, a woman reaches her target heart rate (a concept explained in "A Running Program Designed For You") more quickly than a man. If a man and a woman, for example, are running side by side, he may be comfortably within his target heart rate range, but she may be exceeding hers and, as a consequence, overexerting herself.

Other things may also account for this cardiovascular training difference between a woman and a man. Few women are accustomed to running. In the past, most women gave up strenuous physical activities when they entered adolescence while most men remained active through adolescence. Whether this difference is still a significant factor several years later is open to question. Dr. Kenneth Cooper maintains that "a heart is a heart, lungs are lungs, blood vessels are blood vessels. They have no sex, and the effect on all is the same." Still, any woman who has not remained physically active should be especially careful about not exceeding her target heart rate.

That's one bit of special advice. Here's another. If you are pregnant, jogging can be quite beneficial, at least through the sixth month of pregnancy. But after the sixth month, don't even try to jog. We hardly need to emphasize that you should check with your obstetrician before you start a running program.

Getting Started

If you are not pregnant but eventually hope to be, jogging is an excellent way to prepare your body for pregnancy according to most physicians. A family health report from the U. S. Drug and Health Administration says that the firming effect which jogging has on the muscles of the abdomen and back makes delivery less painful. After delivery the abdomen regains its former shape much sooner than it otherwise would. Finally, many physicians believe that running can relieve the physical and emotional distress which some women experience during menstrual periods and menopause.

Sharing the Experience

Taking that first running step out in public can be a little traumatic for some beginners. It's a natural reaction. We aren't the runners we once were when we were young and we probably look it. The veterans we see running on the roads and through the parks move so swiftly and smoothly. They're graceful. They make running seem effortless. They're beautiful to watch. And the beginner may think to himself: "And here I am, overweight, struggling, slogging along, huffing and puffing like a steam engine."

If you suspect that behind every tree someone is laughing as you go lumbering by — relax and forget it. In the first place, that's mainly your imagination at work. In the second place, even if it were so, so what? So you have a little stage fright, a little trouble looking like this is duck soup for you. Who doesn't? The feeling doesn't last long anyway. You'll get over it and soon begin to look as if you were born to run. In fact you were, and it won't be long before you're getting from it what it has to offer.

Still, if things like that bother you, don't run alone. Hook up with another runner for company. Then you'll have somebody who can share your frustrations, the aches, the pains, and the pleasures of making real progress. And you can share his or hers.

Getting Started

Running with someone will also help you overcome a certain amount of inertia that you probably will experience in the beginning. It is as hard to form a new habit as it is to break an old one. It is difficult to spend time doing something that may at first feel uncomfortable and make you self-conscious. Doing it with someone else makes it all a lot easier.

If you do not have a willing friend, neighbor, husband, or wife for running company, get in touch with your local YMCA or YWCA. Since some kind of running program is usually going on at the Y, it shouldn't be too difficult to find other runners who will be grateful for a little company themselves. Another possible way of starting is to join an organized fitness program that includes running. Programs like that monitor your progress over a definite period and you have the benefit of professional guidance until you are ready to manage your own program. Hundreds of jogging and running clubs that give the same help in a less organized way have sprung up all across the country. Look up some of these. The physical education departments of local high schools and colleges may be able to give you a lot of information about such jogging groups near you.

Smoking, Drinking, And Eating

Although quite prepared to embrace a new habit, the potential runner may begin to worry about a few old ones: "If I jog, will I have to quit smoking, and drinking, and eating my favorite foods?" The answer is no, you don't *have* to. But you may find that you *want* to. You may find that by some curious process your addiction to some things simply leaves you. (We make no promises here!)

If you are a smoker and/or a drinker, however, we can tell you that it will probably be difficult to give up these things when you first start to jog. It will be hard enough for you to give up sedentary habits for an active life of exercise without also depriving yourself of pleasures you have keenly enjoyed for years. But

Getting Started

you may find that you become far less attached to them as you become more attached to the pleasures of running. You may want to quit smoking for the simple reason that it is diminishing the pleasure you get from running. If running does nothing else for you, at the very least it will dramatize in no uncertain terms what smoking has been doing to your body. Joe Henderson's formula tells the running smoker's story: "One non-smoker's jog equals three smoker's jogs." The culprit, of course, is the carbon monoxide which the smoker inhales from his tobacco. Once in the bloodstream it attaches itself to the hemoglobin molecules in the blood and prevents them from transporting oxygen throughout the body. This state of affairs produces an oxygen deficiency that cancels out some of the benefits of jogging. So if you are a smoker, face up to the fact that you can expect fewer benefits from running than the non-smoker will enjoy.

If you are a confirmed drinker, the chances are that you won't be giving it up for jogging. But you ought to know some of the effects it can have on your conditioning. Like smoking, it hampers the distribution of oxygen to the heart, tissues, and muscles. Since alcohol restricts the absorption of the B vitamins, you could end up with a vitamin deficiency if you don't replace these and other nutrients that enable the liver to detoxify the effects of alcohol in the body. Although even competitive runners imbibe now and then and have been known to guzzle beer during their marathon runs, we recommend that you do not run if you have been drinking. Besides putting an undue strain on your heart, alcohol, as you undoubtedly know, can affect your judgment of speed, distance, and your own endurance. Consequently, if you run after you have been drinking, you could harm yourself by overexertion. Even if you insist on dragging yourself out of bed for a jog after a night on the town, it probably won't do you much good anyway. The alcohol will still be in your system, you will tend to tire quickly, and you will end up with a very unsatisfactory run.

Now about food. There are runners who have pet theories about the ideal diet and runners who just have bad eating habits. Wilma Rudolph ate hot dogs, hamburgers, and drank soda pop, and managed to become a champion runner. Some runners swear by a vegetarian diet. Others fill themselves up

Getting Started

with carbohydrates before a race. The best advice we can give about diet is the same advice nutritionists give: eat regularly; eat sensibly; eat a variety of foods — meat, dairy products, cereals, vegetables, and fruit — that will give you the protein, fats, carbohydrates, vitamins, and minerals the body needs for health. Avoid foods such as sugar that have no nutritional value. It furnishes calories for energy, but little else. Get the calories you need from other food.

There are no rules on how you should accommodate your eating schedule to your running program, or vice versa. Some doctors recommend that you wait an hour or two after eating before you set out to run. Others say that it is not necessary for you to wait that long. To be safe, it's a good idea to wait one hour. You do not really have to worry too much about replenishing the calories you consume during your running exercise. Your body will quietly let you know when it needs more fuel. You'll get hungry.

Hunger is just one of many personal messages your body will be sending you in your running program. Your program should be flexible enough to accommodate itself to those messages. As you get acquainted with your body and the ways it reacts to running, you will find that you can pace yourself in a way that suits your body, while steadily improving your fitness.

When, Where, And How To Run

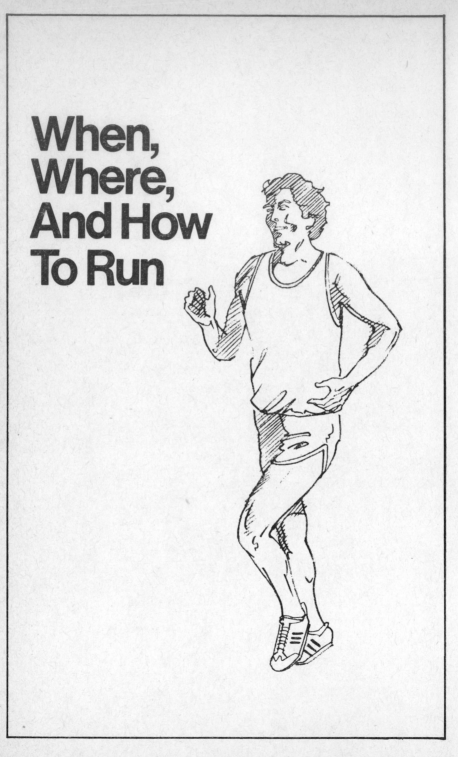

When, Where, And How

IF YOU have ever watched a film of a runner shown in slow motion and studied the intense concentration in his eyes and the way every muscle in his body works together in rippling harmony, driving his body toward the tape, you'll get some idea of what we mean when we talk about true discipline. It's something that comes from the inside. It's never imposed from outside. And you can't do difficult things without it.

The busy executive who loves his work does not sit at his desk wheeling and dealing and talking to three different people on different phones because he's under somebody else's orders. He does it because he wants to. He finds the excitement and the challenge intellectually and emotionally satisfying. He doesn't wake up every morning with a snarl, wishing it were 5 o'clock on Friday afternoon. He looks forward to a day at his desk, knowing that's where he can accomplish his goals, whatever they may be. And one of his most intense pleasures is accomplishing them. Those inner needs and the pleasure of having them satisfied produce their own discipline.

Most of you probably believe that all the things we say about the benefits of running are true. The problem comes in moving from belief to action — from wishing to doing.

Whatever reasons people have for taking up jogging in the first place, those who put up with the initial pains and burdens of becoming runners usually stick it out because it has finally turned out to be fun. It pleases them immensely. Usually it pleases them so much and becomes so necessary that it bothers them to miss a day of it. All you have to do is ask a seasoned runner. It's the rare bird who will not confess being hooked on it. It's a form of play, like any sport. Golf, tennis, boating, handball, and skiing are all sports that people naturally regard as sources of great pleasure. Most people don't think twice about whether they are "good for you." They are all "games" of one kind or another, and for most people games are fun.

Running is really no different. But in the past it has been regarded as being different, the private reserve of oddballs with some special kind of "calling." This view of running as a peculiar kind of vocation reserved for youngsters who are fast on their feet is, we are happy to report, old hat. Running is, purely and simply, a sport and a game like any other. So don't approach running with the thought: "I am about to engage in a special kind of exercise" or "This running thing will be good for me." Running will be good for you, better than any other game we've mentioned — or failed to mention. But that's not the way to think about it. If you do, it is likely that it will not please you, in spite of all those solid benefits we never tire of talking about. And the chances are that you will give it up before it can begin to please you.

If, however, you aren't stuck with an archaic way of thinking about running and really want to take it up for fun, then here's how to go about it.

The first thing you have to do is get yourself a pair of good running shoes. We'll help you with that in a later chapter. Then, to really start yourself on a regular program, you'll have to decide *when* to run.

The Best
Time Of Day

It's important to establish a routine for yourself, geared to your own disposition and living habits. Some runners prefer to run early in the morning, some even before daybreak. They seem to like the solitude available at that hour, when the streets are still empty of traffic and people, and they can slowly get their minds and bodies going and do a little thinking in the silence. And if they are running where they have access to the horizon, they can savor the exhilarating sight of dawn.

That's the poetry of running in the morning. But, alas, it has its prosaic side. If you are not particularly interested in being exhilarated at that time of the morning and you have to be at work by 9 o'clock and it takes you an hour to commute, then, of course, you will have to crawl out of bed at an ungodly hour several days a week so you can get in your running time. That

When, Where, And How

means that you will probably have to forego the late, late show on TV — that is, if you don't want to fall asleep at the office. When you are into a solid running schedule, sleep is one thing you should not stint on, even though you may feel so charged with energy that you think you don't need as much as before.

If you do run before work, it is probably a good idea to eat breakfast beforehand so your body has the fuel it needs for the run. The experts give no iron-clad rules. Dr. Kenneth Cooper finds that runners do very well if they run before they eat. Others prescribe a light, nutritious meal prior to running. You might try both ways and see how you feel. If you choose to eat beforehand, wait a reasonable length of time (about one hour) to allow your body to do its digestive work before giving it other chores to perform.

Some runners are shrewd — and courageous — enough to kill two birds with one stone. They get their exercise in while "commuting" to work. They run to work. Among the most famous of those commuters-by-foot is Senator William Proxmire of Wisconsin, who runs the four or five miles between his home and Capitol Hill at least one way nearly every day.

That can pose a minor problem: the need for a change of clothing once you get to the office. Some runners carry clothes in a small backpack, but that can leave you looking like you slept all night in your suit — not the happiest of impressions to make at the office. Others, with access to locker facilities, keep a change of clothing on the job.

The problem of showering after sweating your way to work cannot be ignored. The issues involved are, to say the least, delicate. And there are too many variables for generalizations to be useful: How hot is it? How far is it to your work? What kind of work do you do? Do you work outside or inside? How casual are your surroundings at work? Are showers available? If there are no showers, how much privacy do you have for a sponge bath? And so on.

People who do their running in the morning say that it sets them up for the day. They are more alert and less likely to become upset by the pressures and frustrations of their work, and at the end of the day they feel less fatigued.

Some people skip lunch and use the time to run at noon. (Check with your doctor before deciding to skip a meal.) It gets them out of the office or house and into a refreshing midday break.

Other runners, however, wait until they have left their work, put their jobs behind them, and headed home. A run at this time provides a nice transition for them, a time to work off some of the tensions that may have built up during the day so that they don't carry them into family life.

Late in the evening seems to appeal to some runners as the best time to work out. The only thing we'd like to say about this choice is that you should end your run at least an hour before you retire. Otherwise you may find it difficult to fall asleep. Running "wakes up" your body in the evening just as effectively as it does in the morning, and it usually takes at least an hour to come down from that peak.

Well, by now it should be clear that *when* you run is an individual thing. Run any time it suits you. If you are a morning person and like to get up with the larks, run in the morning. But if you're the sort who spends most of the morning groping about, don't force yourself to greet the dawn. Leave it to the larks. Run later in the day, when it fits in with *your* metabolism and idiosyncrasies. If you are fortunate enough to be on top of things at either end of the day, the possibilities you have for selecting a running time are simply multiplied.

Establish
A Routine

Once you have decided on the best time for you to run, stick to it! If on one day you run in the morning, the next day in mid-afternoon, and the third in the evening, you are not building a strong routine. You should be striving to develop a new habit of exercise, and this is much easier to do if you exercise at the same time every day. Any habit is largely a conditioned reflex. And conditioned reflexes come about through repetition. The repetition develops a patterned response in our minds and bodies. If something interrupts this pattern, most of us become very uncomfortable.

At one time or another, all of us have felt great distress about a simple thing like not having our newspaper delivered. We feel like skinning the newsboy alive. Our habit of reading the paper every day has been interrupted. But it's more complicated than that. We were used to reading it at a particular time, say after a good dinner, and the pattern of contentment associated with it may also be disturbed.

Most running programs, including our own, ask you to run three times a week as a minimum requirement. This helps reinforce the habit of running, but its main purpose is to develop cardiovascular conditioning through frequent running. But *more* is not necessarily better. Experts in physical fitness tend to agree that running days should alternate with days of rest, since rest for the body is as much a part of developing fitness as exercise. Don't for example, run on three successive days and then take the other four days off. Space your runs so that you have rest days in between.

Bill Bowerman, track coach at the University of Oregon, a school famous for its distance runners, trains his teams this way. He calls it the "hard-easy method" — a day of hard work followed by a day of easy work or rest.

When Not To Run

Recommended schedules should be followed as faithfully as possible, but not blindly. There are certain times when you have no business running. If, for example, you have the flu, a cold, or some other ailment, don't overexert yourself and possibly harm your body by trying to run. If you feel a cold coming on, however, running may help you get rid of it. But if you try this cure, follow Dr. Kostrubala's recommendations. He suggests that you dress warmly, take two aspirin in a glass of milk, and then go out for a run. Jog slowly and see how you feel. Continue jogging until your body grows warm, even hot. Then try to keep your temperature at that level. When you get home, drink hot coffee or tea with honey if you like. Soak for awhile in a hot bath and take a nap for a few hours. When you wake up, Dr. Kostrubala suggests, your cold may have disappeared. If it has not, don't fight it. Let it run its course.

Don't run when you have been drinking. Some runners say you should not run when you are suffering with a hangover; others say running is the best cure there is for a hangover, simple weariness, or lack of sleep. On the other hand, some runners recommend that you not run if you are overtired. We would tend to agree with this. As we said earlier in this chapter, when you are running you should get as much sleep as you can manage with your schedule. But when it comes to strong differences over borderline questions of this sort, the person who really has the answer in specific cases is the runner himself.

Where To Run

Where you choose to run is another individual matter and the range of choices is obviously unlimited. Well, at least unlimited as far as space is concerned. Just look around you — nothing but spaces to run through. Just pick a route. Maybe you're lucky enough to live in a town that offers not just running space — every place has that — but different kinds of spaces to make your running as interesting as possible. You'll have your favorites and you'll probably discover new ones every week, but in making these discoveries you should always consider safety.

Traffic must always be taken into account. And you don't have to be a genius to realize that some city areas are just not safe enough to run through at any hour. The best way to protect yourself against these possible dangers is to check over the routes you plan to use beforehand.

When, Where, And How

When you are choosing a route, pay close attention to the surface. A lot of joggers say grass is the very best surface for jogging. It is springy and comfortable. It cushions your feet and ankles, knees, and other joints against sprains and aches. City dwellers can usually find some strip of grass or other unpaved area to run on, even if it is only the boulevard along your street. Try the edges of cemeteries and reservoirs. Parks and forest preserves are among the most ideal areas for runners. But grass can be deceptive. You can be loping along at a nice, even pace. Then wham! It turns out that that nice smooth grassy surface is not so nice and smooth after all. It is filled with little valleys and hills, imperceptible holes, tiny bumps. Any one of these can surprise you, throw you off stride, and strain ligaments and tendons that are probably bearing as much stress as they can already.

Grass that grows in sun-baked soil can also be deceptive and dangerous, according to Jack Batten, author of *The Complete Jogger*. He reports an incident that occurred at the Amateur Athletic Union championship marathon held at Belmont, California, when many runners dropped out of the race with twisted ankles after only two miles. The cause: hard-baked earth that was both bumpy and unresilient. Even shoes especially chosen to compensate for the poor condition of the ground did not protect the runners. So when you're going to run on unpaved surfaces and you are not familiar with the terrain, keep a watchful eye on the ground.

If you can't find a nice springy, green surface in your area to use, pavement is the alternative. It may be harder than grass, but it is not so tricky. It is usually smooth and consistent. And if there are breaks in the sidewalk you can usually spot them far enough ahead so you don't break your rhythm and/or ankle suddenly. One good thing about pavement — you don't have to travel far to find it. But it does have its drawbacks. Most foot and leg problems are either caused or aggravated by running on hard surfaces like concrete or asphalt. You can compensate for this somewhat by wearing good, shock-absorbing running shoes. Learn to spring forward lightly when you are running on hard surfaces to avoid the painful jarring effects of pavement. And if you insist on using the street instead of the sidewalk, be on the alert for cars. Even if you wear reflective strips on your clothing, you may not be seen by a motorist; you should run as you drive — defensively.

Jack Batten has some useful advice for city runners — to make your run pleasant even though you are not surrounded by trees and grass and country smells. Find an old residential area with beautiful homes and meandering streets that can occupy your attention while you run. Keep away from high-rise apartment complexes unless you want to use up all your energy battling the winds they generate. Stay away from traffic lights and congested areas where there are a lot of pedestrians. They can cause you to lose momentum and break your stride because you will be concerned about collisions. And watch out for curbs. Drive around and plan out your running course ahead of time, arranging it so that you run roughly in a circle. That way you will end up back where you started. In city running be particularly watchful for dogs.

There are some things to watch out for if you plan to jog in the country, too. Make sure you are not trespassing on someone's land. Get a map and check out the locale first, so you know where you are going. You want to be careful that you do not get carried away by the beauties of nature, the song of the birds, the clean air — and get lost. And since you do not want to end up miles away from your car at the end of your run, plan a route that will bring you back to your starting point.

Some further precautions: If you are jogging in an isolated area, be aware of what could happen — a twisted ankle, or a pulled muscle. You may be miles from your car and help.

Use common sense in hilly country. You use more oxygen when you run uphill, so slow down. Don't overwork those muscles and lungs that are used to flat surfaces.

Weather

In this world there are cities and areas that have ideal jogging conditions year round, but the chances are better than good that you are not living in one of them. The ideal jogging conditions are a windless day with the thermometer hovering in the

When, Where, And How

neighborhood of 50 F (10 C). But what do you do when icicles are forming, a gale threatens to blow you off the path and turn your running into flying, or the heat makes you feel like your shoes are going to melt?

Cold-Weather Running

Cold weather does not present any serious problems for you, especially if you are in reasonably good condition. If you have heart problems, however, ask your doctor if it is okay for you to brave very cold weather even if he has already permitted you to run. High wind-chill factors are the greatest threats to you in cold weather, since you can suffer frostbite if you are not adequately protected from the wind. You must remember that when you run, your own motion against the wind increases the wind-chill factor and increases the risk of frostbite. Be sure all normally exposed areas of skin are covered: head, face, ears, and hands. A wind-chill chart can be found at the back of this book. Understand it and use it as a guide. If you are wearing proper clothing, only the bitterest cold should bother you. The important thing to remember is that you must dress in layers in order to create your own insulation.

The following articles of clothing are recommended for cold weather. Obviously you would use all, or any combination, of these as required by weather conditions: cotton shorts; wool fishnet underwear; long underwear; turtleneck shirt; wool or nylon warm-up pants; a long-sleeved hooded sweatshirt (fleece-lined cotton or wool); a windbreaker (preferably cotton poplin, so that sweat will evaporate without condensing inside); two pairs of socks; leather or nylon running shoes (waterproof, of course); mittens (they keep you warmer than gloves); a hat or cap (your body loses more heat through your head than anywhere else); and, the finishing touch, a wool or nylon ski mask to cover your head and face. With this outfit you should be ready to face any very cold day.

When you run in cold weather, beware of ice on the road, and remember to taper off your run slowly so you will not catch a chill. When you arrive home, change out of your damp, sweaty clothes right away.

When, Where, And How

Hot-Weather Running

When it is hot, be especially careful. Cut down on your usual program or stop altogether. Dr. Kenneth Cooper says to stop running when the thermometer hits 98 F. Dr. Terence Kavanagh tells his heart-patient joggers to quit if it gets warmer than 85 F. But for safety's sake it is best to lower even these limits a bit. If you are just starting to run or if you have heart problems, if you are overweight or are more than 40 years old, you had better set 80 to 85 F as your temperature limit (especially if the humidity is high). When you do run, wear a hat of some kind to protect you from the sun.

When you run in hot weather, your blood pressure can drop dangerously or you could suffer heat exhaustion. If you start feeling dizzy and dehydrated while jogging and your pulse and breathing grow very rapid, you could very well be on your way to heat exhaustion. *Stop exercising immediately.* Get out of the sun, drink fluids (tepid, not cold), and rest. If symptoms continue, call your doctor.

Running in heat also slows down the blood circulation, placing a greater burden on your heart. And, of course, you will sweat a lot more so your body loses more water than usual. To replace it, drink a full glass of water before you start and one every 15 or 20 minutes during your run. A few pinches of salt dissolved in the water will help. But if your stomach is empty, omit the salt or it will probably cause stomach cramps. Wearing a fishnet vest will also help by creating an insulating layer of air next to your body, reducing the temperature.

An important thing to remember about heat is that it takes your body about two weeks to adjust. So take it easy and let your body tell you when it's ready to go under the changed conditions.

Wind, Rain, and Altitude

If you run in a strong wind, you are going to be expending six percent more oxygen than you would under ordinary conditions. So, if you are running in a stiff breeze, slow down and you will get the same benefit as you would from a faster run. When you set out to run on a windy day, start with the wind in front of you at the beginning of your workout; then at the end, when you are more tired, you will have it at your back, helping to push you along.

Rain need not be a deterrent unless you're afraid of melting, but you will need some protection. Wear waterproof outer clothes, of course, and as many layers as you need to keep warm. Don't linger in them after the run but get into dry things as soon as you get home.

High altitudes are a source of special problems. When you get to 5000 feet above sea level and beyond, it takes a lot more time for oxygen to be absorbed into your blood and travel throughout your body. So your heart has to work a lot harder at its job. Plan on taking at least four to six weeks to get adjusted to a new high altitude, and adapt your jogging routine accordingly. Most runners recommend cutting your program by about 50% at the beginning. If you find yourself short of breath, even at that rate, slow down even more.

Running Indoors

Indoor running is the best solution for running in bad or extreme weather conditions but it does have drawbacks. While there are no bumps or potholes, cars, or pedestrians to worry about, running indoors, going around and around and around the same track, can become boring after a while. If you're trying to run a mile, it may take you 20 or more laps to make it. Your mind tends to grow numb, and it is easy to become discouraged. The evidence shows that people who habitually run only on indoor tracks are the most likely to give up the sport.

Jack Batten's advice to them is to switch directions every other day. By running counter-clockwise one day and clockwise the next you will also help avoid some orthopedic problems that could result from constantly running on a surface that slopes in one direction. By changing your running direction you vary, in effect, the slope of the banked turns. It is also a good idea to carry a lap counter with you. That way you won't have to remember how far you've run. The counter will tell you.

Starting
Your Program

Now that you're ready to run, remember: Don't begin without a plan — one that puts you on a regular running program. You'll find such a plan in the next chapter, one that is flexible enough for runners of all ages and different physical conditions.

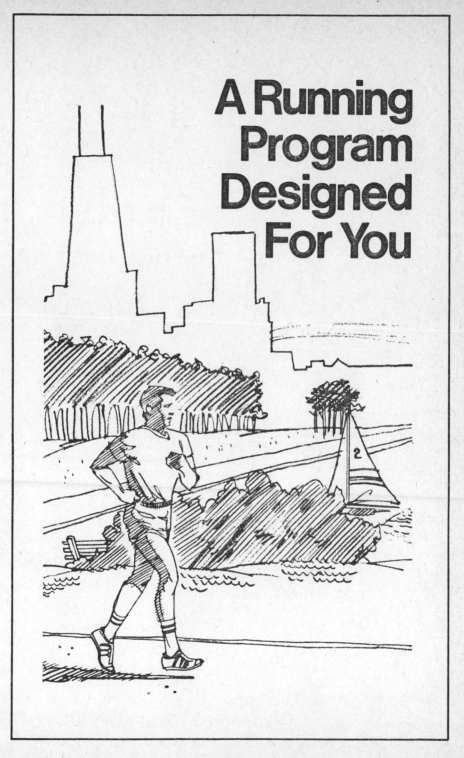

A Running Program Designed For You

Your Own Program

ONLY A FEW years ago, if you thought about runners at all, you thought about stadiums and oval tracks with precisely chalked lanes, roaring crowds, and lean, long-legged people with numbers on their backs, shaking their muscles loose before crouching down into the blocks. Real physical fitness was something you associated with athletes who trained for it under special coaches. If you saw someone running down the street in your neighborhood, you figured he was either a thief or a member of the local high-school track squad. If he looked too innocent to be a thief and too old to be in school, you probably regarded him as just a little strange.

Now, you probably accept the presence of dozens of people racing through the neighborhood. You may give them room to go sailing by but not much thought, except to feel a little envy that "there but for my inertia go I." If the number of people who have overcome that inertia continues growing at the present rate, another thought might pop into your head — "I must be missing something terrific."

That's not too far-fetched, since in the past few years the value of running has been spreading as fast as juicy gossip. But the "gossip" is based on scientific facts and it isn't being passed along on the sly. Tips, techniques, guidelines, and formal programs on running have flourished by word of mouth and in the pages of newsletters, papers, magazines, and books. The advocates of running number in the millions in the United States alone. And the slim ranks of track coaches have swelled to an army of therapists, physicians, and "evangelical" runners who are "coaching" people to better health.

It turns out that the slightly strange 40-year-old who used to lope through your neighborhood probably knew what he was up to all the time. It's only lately that we have come to understand what he's doing, chiefly through people like Sheehan, Fixx, Ullyot, Cooper, Kostrubala, and Bowerman — names nearly as well known in the world of running as those of great runners like Paavo Nurmi and Frank Shorter — who have developed running programs based on solid physiological and medical facts. Despite their differences, all these programs are designed to help you become a runner.

Running Programs

Before people like Cooper, Fixx, and the others came along, you probably would have had to do a little digging to come up with guidelines for an organized running program, once you had decided to put a little more action into your life. Now the new runner faces the problem of choosing which program to follow, for they vary considerably. One may be quite formal and meticulously organized, while another is casual and loosely structured. Still others might be part of larger programs of physical exercise that include many different kinds of activity.

Too often, these programs tend to frighten off even the bravest soul. It is hard enough just deciding to leave the completely sedentary life behind once and for all. Now, having made the decision and picked a program, you find yourself staring at pages that ask you to perform deeds that seem rather formidable, like running two miles when you haven't exercised in ten years. Or running a one-mile course at a speed which seems roughly equivalent to that of an impala who has just spotted a lion with a hungry look bearing down on him.

Programs like this, so good in themselves, can appear too forbidding even to the best-intentioned individual and, as a consequence, turn off a great many potential runners at the outset. Even if the build-up to more strenuous exertion is gradual, the thought of eventually running several miles or more within 30 or even 60 minutes appears to be an impossible dream, stuff for Don Quixotes tilting with 100-foot windmills. The struggle hardly seems worth the aches and pains. Better to go back to slouching in a chair.

Goals like these seem unattainable. The truth is, however, that they can be reached. And there is no need to be frightened off if your program allows you to accomplish goals like these at your own pace. As imposing as achievements of this order may seem, your body is able to develop the conditioning and endurance to make them possible. As you progress comfortably in

Your Own Program

your running program, what may have once seemed "unnatural" and extreme for the condition of your body becomes a natural and exhilarating activity.

We at CONSUMER GUIDE® and our consultants in medicine, physical fitness, and health have studied all the standard and currently popular exercise programs. We evaluated them from a variety of viewpoints. Our findings were recently published in the book, *Rating the Exercises,* by the Editors of CONSUMER GUIDE® (New York, William Morrow & Co.). The exercise programs covered in that study were classified into those which are intended primarily to tone up the body's muscular structure and increase physical strength and agility, and those designed to improve the functioning of the heart and respiratory — that is, the cardiovascular — systems of the body. Our study concluded that the best form of exercise is one that contributes to the fitness of the heart and lungs, a finding in agreement with those of the American Heart Association, the American College of Sports Medicine, and other important groups. Men do not die because they lack the rippling pectoral muscles of an Arnold Schwarzenegger, nor do women go to premature graves because they lack the solid curves of Racquel Welch's figure. Most of them die because their two power plants — the heart and the pulmonary system — degenerate to such an extent that they break down years earlier than they ought to. This breakdown is responsible for more premature deaths than all other diseases put together.

A second conclusion our experts came to is that running is among the best of all exercises to prevent this breakdown.

Many of the running programs we examined are excellent for this purpose. These include Dr. Cooper's aerobics program, the President's Council on Physical Fitness guide, the official YMCA exercise program, and the techniques recommended by experts like George Sheehan, Thaddeus Kostrubala, William Bowerman, James Fixx, and others.

But some of them can be quite demanding and may call for a degree of commitment that many of you simply are not prepared to give, either because of time or your lifestyle. So, drawing upon the soundest principles of cardiovascular conditioning, we at CONSUMER GUIDE® have devised a running program that demands enough to get the job done, but is flexible enough for you to adapt it to your personal needs, age, present level of fitness, and lifestyle.

We do not want to scare you off or ask more of you than you can reasonably do. We want to get you started, keep you going, and help you finally experience the physical, mental, and emotional exhilaration — and, best of all, the well-being — that comes from running with ease. That euphoric "high" we talked about awaits you. We want you to share that with us.

And here is one of the simplest and surest ways to do it.

The Consumer Guide®
Running Program

The aim of our running program is very simple: to condition your heart and lungs and strengthen them through the most effective exercise for that purpose we know of — running. Briefly summarized, in this running program you will be taking yourself through four levels of conditioning, with progressive stages of conditioning at each level. The conditioning goals are met naturally and automatically as you progress through the program. The most important thing about it is that you advance easily and comfortably, in step with your own body's demands.

Earlier we described the heart and respiratory systems as two power plants that drive our bodies. They might be better described as two systems in a single power plant. One depends on the other. And the rest of the body depends on both. In the simplest terms, the lungs take in the oxygen the body needs to "burn" food, which is the body's fuel. As in any burning process, waste gases are given off in the form of carbon dioxide. A transport system is needed to carry the oxygen from the lungs to the cells and then carry off the waste carbon dioxide. The blood vessels and the heart provide that transport system, a complicated arrangement of pipes and a simple yet extraordinary pump. If the lungs take in less oxygen than the transport system should deliver, the body's cells are deprived of oxygen

Your Own Program

they need. And if, on the other hand, the heart and blood cannot transport oxygen as fast as the lungs can take it in, the same deprivation occurs. Obviously, if both systems are crippled, the cells suffer even more.

So any worthwhile physical fitness program must focus on these two systems and their mutual dependence. According to the American Heart Association's Committee on Exercise and Fitness and the American College of Sports Medicine, an exercise contributes to cardiovascular fitness only if it involves both systems and is sustained for at least 15 minutes and preferably for 20 minutes or more. This is why a game of tennis, even a spirited one, is not the most useful exercise for strengthening the heart and lungs. There may be periods of furious activity, full of lunging and running and rapid starts and stops. But they are too short and there's too much rest in between. The action is not sustained action, the kind that makes a long-distance jog of 20 or 30 minutes one of the most effective exercises for the cardiovascular system.

Our running program, like a lot of others, is based on this principle of sustained action. But most programs set distance or speed as the basic goal in generating this sustained action. The CONSUMER GUIDE® program, on the other hand, is unique in establishing the time period for running as the basic goal. The length of the exercise in minutes of sustained action is the crucial element of the program. How far or how fast you run is up to you. The program is structured to enable each of you to proceed at your own pace through successive stages according to a personal timetable. When you are ready to move ahead, you do. If you are not ready to go to a higher level of conditioning, you wait until you are.

Your Target Heart Rate

The conditioning effects of sustained action organized into a series of gradually increasing time spans depend on an important biological fact. Everyone has what is called a "maximum heart rate," generally based on age and current physical condition. A person's maximum heart rate is the number of beats his heart makes per minute when his body is undergoing maximum

Your Own Program

Your Target Heart Rate and Heart Rate Range

Maintaining your target heart rate is the key to the CONSUMER GUIDE® running program. Your maximum heart rate is the greatest number of beats per minute that your heart is capable of. During exercise, your heart rate should be approximately 75% of this maximum. To obtain the cardiovascular benefits of running — or of any other exercise — you maintain a heart rate between 70% and 85% of your maximum, for at least 15 and preferably for 20 minutes. If your heart rate is less than 70% of the maximum you will not improve your cardiovascular condition. If it exceeds 85% of your maximum, you are overdoing and should relax your pace.

Age	Your Maximum Heart Rate	Your Target Heart Rate (75% Of The Maximum)	Your Target Heart Rate Range (Between 70% And 85% Of The Maximum)
20	200 beats per minute	150 beats per minute	140 to 170 beats per minute
25	195 beats per minute	146 beats per minute	137 to 166 beats per minute
30	190 beats per minute	142 beats per minute	133 to 162 beats per minute
35	185 beats per minute	139 beats per minute	130 to 157 beats per minute
40	180 beats per minute	135 beats per minute	126 to 153 beats per minute
45	175 beats per minute	131 beats per minute	123 to 149 beats per minute
50	170 beats per minute	127 beats per minute	119 to 145 beats per minute
55	165 beats per minute	124 beats per minute	116 to 140 beats per minute
60	160 beats per minute	120 beats per minute	112 to 136 beats per minute
65	155 beats per minute	116 beats per minute	109 to 132 beats per minute
70	150 beats per minute	112 beats per minute	105 to 128 beats per minute

Your Own Program

exertion. Your maximum heart rate will generally be 220 beats per minute, minus your age. If you are 20 years old, your maximum heart rate will be 200. If you are 60, it will be 160. This formula is derived from the observation that for each year you live your heart loses about a beat a minute.

The "target heart rate," as it is called in cardiovascular exercise programs, is pegged at around 70% to 85% of your maximum heart rate. Everyone's heart and overall physiology is different, so the target heart rate of individuals is normally described as falling within a target heart rate range. The accompanying chart gives the maximum heart rate, the target heart rate range, and the target heart rate for ages 20 through 70 in five-year increments. You can calculate your own rates and range from this if your age falls between the ages listed.

Your target heart rate is the key to conditioning, and using it in the CONSUMER GUIDE® running program is simplicity itself. In the program outlined later, each conditioning level contains six time stages. Each stage calls for sustained exercise for a specific period of time, and as you move from one stage to the next, the period of sustained exercise increases.

This is where the target heart rate range comes in: *regardless of the stage you are in at any given time, you should maintain your heartbeat somewhere within your target heart rate range while you are exercising to achieve the conditioning results you desire.*

Just as it is important to reach your target rate, it is vital not to exceed it. If you find that you are reaching 90% or more of your maximum heart rate, you are overdoing. Slow down or drop back to the previous stage. Remember that you should "train, not strain." How do you go about doing this? Simple. Take your pulse while you are exercising. Of course, it isn't necessary to do this on the run. All you have to do is stop after you have been running for a bit and check it to see where you are.

How To Take Your Pulse

You can determine if you are within your target heart rate range by placing three fingers over the artery near the center of your

Your Own Program

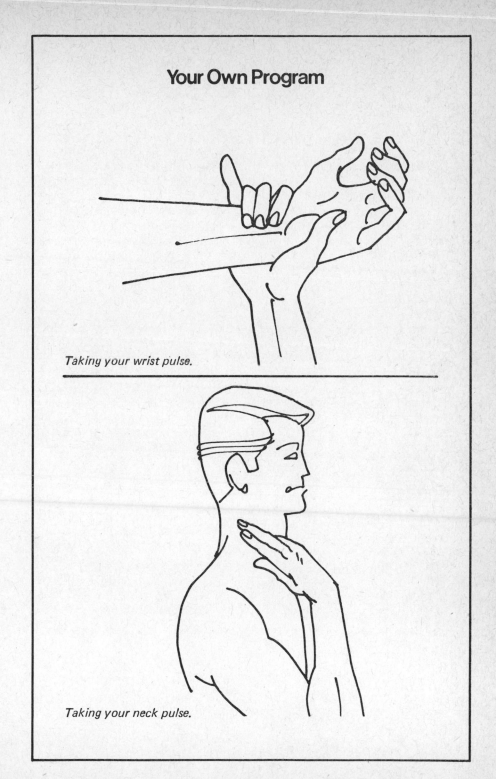

Taking your wrist pulse.

Taking your neck pulse.

Your Own Program

wrist. Touch three fingers lightly to that area until you can feel the pulse. Using a stopwatch or the second hand on a wristwatch or clock, count the number of pulses for a period of 15 seconds. Then multiply this number by four to give you your heart rate in beats per minute.

If you have difficulty in locating the pulse in your wrist — nothing to be alarmed about — you can find your heart rate by placing two or three fingers along your neck about one inch below the top of your jawbone and going through the same procedure.

Benefits You Can Expect From Running

Running produces mental and physical results. Your cardio-vascular system will be improved and, in all likelihood, your general well-being enhanced. The benefits you can expect are, of course, determined by the amount of time you devote to running and the length of time you maintain your target heart rate.

Duration of Sustained Exercise	Frequency	Benefits
15 to 30 minutes	3 times per week	You will meet minimum standards of physical fitness
30 to 40 minutes	4 times per week	Your body fat will be reduced and your physical condition improved
40 to 60 minutes	4 times per week	Cholesterol and triglyceride (fat) levels will be reduced
60 minutes or more	3 times per week	You may experience the runner's "high"

Your Own Program

Once you have determined that you are comfortable within the range of your target heart rate, you simply have to maintain the level of your exercise. You want to be sure that you stay within the range of your target rate and as close as possible to the target rate itself. It will take a little experimenting at first, but after a while you will be able to tell if you are within your range by the way you feel.

If you are tiring quickly or noticeably and you are exercising within your target rate range, you should reassess your range and lower it. Slow down until you are still working hard but not overextending yourself. If, on the other hand, you do not feel the effects of your running, it is likely you are not exercising up to your target rate.

Before we get to the program, you might be interested in the benefits that can be derived from this running program, according to Charles Kuntzleman, well-known physical fitness expert and national consultant to the YMCA on matters of exercise and physical fitness. The chart assumes that the sustained exercise is performed at a level of intensity within the target heart range of the individual.

Now you are ready to begin. We trust that you have heeded our advice about having a medical examination before beginning any running program. Your doctor has given you the go-ahead and you want to get running. Do remember, though, that if at any point in your exercise you suffer from a severe shortness of breath, dizziness, lightheadedness, nausea, or experience tightness or pains in the chest, stop exercising immediately. And report these warning symptoms to your physician.

Level 1: Beginning Your Program

Here is the base on which you will build: a good brisk walk in the fresh air. Level 1 is the breaking-in period. After all, your body

Your Own Program

Level 1: Beginning Your Program

Level 1 is your introduction to the exciting world of the runner. A program of brisk walks will get your body in shape for the time when you actually start to run. Walking is also a beneficial cardiovascular exercise, one mild enough for almost everyone to enjoy. As your physical condition improves, try more challenging walks: cover a greater distance or walk uphill. This will enable you to maintain your target heart rate.

Stage	Duration of Exercise	Frequency	Activity
1	15 minutes	3 or 4 times per week	Walk
2	17 minutes	3 or 4 times per week	Walk
3	20 minutes	3 or 4 times per week	Walk
4	23 minutes	3 or 4 times per week	Walk
5	26 minutes	3 or 4 times per week	Walk
6	30 minutes	3 or 4 times per week	Walk

has been stagnating through long years of relative disuse and needs to be prepared for the rigors of running that lie ahead. Your feet, your legs, your back — your whole body, really — and your cardiovascular system in particular are about to do things they haven't done for years and you want to make it as easy as possible for them.

You will want to walk as briskly as it takes to get your heart rate up to its target and continue at that rate for the times specified in the chart. You should progress through the specified time stages as you feel capable of doing it. Whenever

Your Own Program

you feel comfortable moving from the 15-minute stage 1 to the 17-minute stage 2, make the change.

If you feel daring and want to make any substantial jump ahead to a later stage, you should bear in mind all the cautions we have raised about trying to do too much too soon. It is all too tempting for us to imagine ourselves as being younger and more limber than we really are. It's nice to overestimate what we can do in some things. It even helps us carry it off. But in exercise, it's not a very good idea. Still, some of you will really be conditioned enough to move ahead quickly. Some, in fact, will find themselves prepared to either skim through Level 1 or skip it altogether and begin at Level 2. Don't do it, however, unless your physician tells you it is okay for you to begin at an advanced level.

It is best to arrange your exercise days with intervening days for rest whenever possible. If you arrange your program by the week, this is easily done. If you are exercising four times a week, however, two of your exercise days will be consecutive.

Level 2: Starting To Run

Now you will begin to run, at least part of the time. Level 2 extends the times assigned to each stage and intensifies the exercise. We recommend that within each stage you alternate walking with jogging. While this is the basic pattern for this level, the ideal would be that by the time you have completed stage 6 of this level you will be conditioned enough to jog non-stop, having eliminated walking altogether. Of course, not everyone will be able to accomplish this. As long as you maintain your target heart rate, it is not important whether you walk as well as jog. Indeed, older people and those with physical limitations may have to continue the walk-jog pattern throughout this level.

The program is made flexible with these differences in mind.

Your Own Program

Level 2: Starting To Run

In Level 2, you add running to your exercise program. Start with a 50:50 ratio of walking to running. As you progress from stage to stage, gradually increase the amount of time you spend running and reduce the time you walk. By the time you reach stage 4, you may run throughout the exercise period. If you wish, you may continue to combine walking and running. Be sure to maintain your target heart rate.

Stage	Duration of Exercise	Frequency	Activity
1	18 minutes	4 times per week	Run/walk/ run/walk
2	20 minutes	4 times per week	Run/walk/ run/walk
3	23 minutes	4 times per week	Run/walk/ run/walk
4	25 minutes	4 times per week	Run or run/ walk/run/walk
5	28 minutes	4 times per week	Run or run/ walk/run/walk
6	30 minutes	4 times per week	Run or run/ walk/run/walk

Use this flexibility to adapt it to yourself. Having gone through six stages of walking in Level 1 and improved your conditioning, simple walking in Level 2 will probably not be enough to maintain your heartbeat within your target range. Now your chief aim will be to gradually increase the proportion of jogging to walking. When you do it is up to you.

A good way of keeping track of your progress is to use the "telephone pole maneuver." You walk from one pole to the

Your Own Program

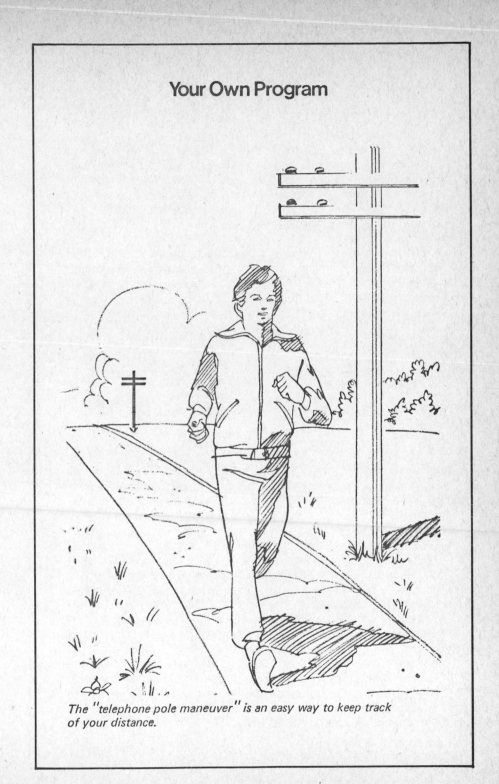

The "telephone pole maneuver" is an easy way to keep track of your distance.

next, jog to the third, walk to the fourth, and so on. You can increase your activity by walking from one pole to the next and then running past the next two. You may want to maintain a certain ratio until you are well on your way through the level, in stage 3 or 4. Your target heart rate and the way you feel will determine what you do. The two, as it turns out, usually send the same message.

At the end of stage 6 you can move to Level 3, which also combines walking and jogging. The only requirement is that you establish a ratio that is comfortable for you and sustains your target heart rate throughout a 30-minute period of exercise.

Level 3: The Accomplished Runner

When you have reached this point in your running program you have reached a level where you have done more than merely maintain your level of physical fitness. You are actually improving it. As your conditioning improves, your cardiovascular system can support the same amount of exertion with a lower heart rate. Put another way, it can deliver the same amount of oxygen to the body's cells as before, while not working as hard at it. This means that in your improved condition, if the intensity of your exercises did not increase, your heartbeat would fall below your target heart rate range. As you proceed through the remaining stages of the program, you will find that you are running harder and faster to maintain your target heart rate and, as a bonus, burning up sufficient calories to slim you down.

If you were able to complete stage 6 of Level 2 with running as your sole exercise, continue that effort through Level 3. Those who feel more comfortable alternating longer periods of jogging with short walks should continue this way if it maintains their heartbeat at their target rate.

Your Own Program

Level 3: The Accomplished Runner

By the time you reach Level 3 you will be a veteran, one of those runners you used to admire. You may run throughout the exercise periods or combine running and walking, whichever is most comfortable for you. If you decide to stay at Level 3 rather than moving on to Level 4, you will continue to strengthen your cardiovascular system as long as you maintain your target heart rate.

Stage	Duration of Exercise	Frequency	Activity
1	33 minutes	4 times per week	Run or run/walk/run/walk
2	35 minutes	4 times per week	Run or run/walk/run/walk
3	38 minutes	4 times per week	Run or run/walk/run/walk
4	40 minutes	4 times per week	Run or run/walk/run/walk
5	43 minutes	4 times per week	Run or run/walk/run/walk
6	45 minutes	4 times per week	Run or run/walk/run/walk

Many runners or runner-walkers might prefer to stay within Level 3 and go no further. There may be several reasons for this. They may not be able to spare the time required in Level 4. Or they may not be interested in longer periods of intense exertion. If for these or other reasons you prefer to remain at Level 3, be assured that you will continue to reap substantial cardiovascular benefits.

Level 4:
The Advanced Runner

This is for the serious runner. If you are able to perform at this level, you are into an advanced stage of running that may reward you with that feeling of euphoria described in an earlier chapter. Those runners who have experienced this "high" in-

---

Level 4: The Advanced Runner

Level 4 is for the dedicated runner, one for whom running is intensely pleasurable. Once you reach stage 6, you may experience the euphoria known as the runner's "high." In any case, you can consider yourself an expert. You may run throughout the exercise periods or combine running with walking as you did earlier.

Stage	Duration of Exercise	Frequency	Activity
1	48 minutes	3 or 4 times per week	Run or run/walk/ run/walk
2	50 minutes	3 or 4 times per week	Run or run/walk/ run/walk
3	53 minutes	3 or 4 times per week	Run or run/walk/ run/walk
4	55 minutes	3 or 4 times per week	Run or run/walk/ run/walk
5	58 minutes	3 or 4 times per week	Run or run/walk/ run/walk
6	60 minutes	3 or 4 times per week	Run or run/walk/ run/walk

variably encounter it after a sustained run of at least 45 minutes, but more often at 60 minutes or more.

The great majority of those who work at Level 4 will be serious runners, running flat out for the entire duration of each stage. However, there is no law banning a relief period of walking if that suits you. As before, the target heart rate must be observed for cardiovascular improvement.

A Final Word

We feel that the CONSUMER GUIDE® running program is not only effective but also easy to live with, an important point in this busy world. You compete with yourself and not against a set of arbitrary standards that may be, for one reason or another, inappropriate for you as an individual. You decide how fast and how far you want to progress, because you are the best judge of your own needs and abilities. As long as you maintain your target heart rate for the periods specified, you can be quite sure your cardiovascular system will benefit. Of course, once you have achieved the level at which you wish to remain, you may find it necessary to increase your speed and/or distance in order to maintain your target heart rate. By this time, however, you will be an accomplished runner, one who thoroughly enjoys this delightful sport.

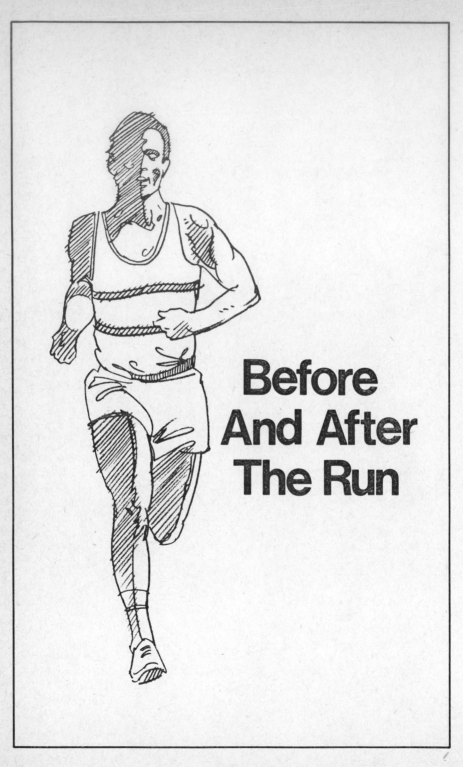

Before And After The Run

Before And After The Run

THERE IS more to running than running. You cannot simply jump into your shoes, set out at a brisk pace, and then relax. Every experienced runner — every experienced athlete — knows the importance of warming up and cooling down.

Warming Up

When we go to a track meet, we go to watch the events. Most of us pay little attention to all the other activities that are going on down on the field. The pole vaulter is doing ten quick push-ups, several racers are jogging leisurely around the track, and others are running in place. Some athletes are doing toe touches, others body twists, still others hurdler's stretches, and still others . . . well, the list is pretty long.

The scene really is a combination of mass calisthenics and jogging. It is not essential or even particularly interesting for us as spectators but it certainly is for the competitors who will run, jump, hurdle, and vault. They know they have to warm up, to get their muscles loosened and limbered, and their hearts and lungs pumping.

This is true for every sport. Football players, tennis players, volleyball players, even serious table tennis players go through various forms of warm-up exercises designed to work on the specific muscles, ligaments, tendons, and joints that will absorb the stress of their particular activity.

It is just as important for the jogger. The jogger needs to be concerned about preparing not only the muscular and skeletal systems but the cardiovascular system as well. In effect, you want to warm up your heart and lungs, to stimulate them and get them ready, because they are going to be used and tested just like the muscles of your legs and the joints of your feet and knees. It only takes five to ten minutes just before the run.

For the runner who is out for the exercise of it, however, or the jogger who has only a limited amount of time before work or before dinner to do his or her few miles, it is tempting to skip the warm-up. After all, it is uninteresting. For us, *running* is the

Before And After The Run

main event but, if we skip this very important element, we often pay for it.

It is estimated that as many as half the injuries caused by running could have been avoided if the runner had warmed up properly. The muscles and the joints are simply not ready to handle serious running unless they are warmed up.

We are not saying this is the greatest cause of runners' aches and pains — you are going to have those anyway — we are talking about the strains and sprains that can be avoided, about injuries that can plague you while you are running as well as those that may force you to curtail your running or even to give it up entirely.

Every jogger, no matter how long he or she has been at it, should warm up before beginning a run. You know how your car reacts when it has been sitting idle for a while, especially in the dead of winter. Well, the human body reacts in much the same way. The body of a regular runner, of course, is more used to the activity. But, even so, it has been at rest since the last run, maybe a day or two before, and the muscles and joints have to be primed once again.

If you are a beginner at running, and let us assume an out-of-condition beginner, you should not go at your warm-up activities too strenuously, or try to do too much at the start. You could very well defeat yourself before you even start to run. As in running itself, you should take an "easy-does-it" approach, warming up at your own pace.

You will want to work primarily on flexibility; that is what enables the various parts of your body to handle the rigors of running. Just as there are limits to how far the knee of a professional football player will bend, there are limitations on the body parts of the jogger — especially in the feet, ankles, and lower legs.

For your overall comfort, however, you should consider the whole body, even your neck, shoulders, and arms. You are not out to tone these muscles, nor is your purpose to give them a real work-out. All you want to do is loosen them up so that they will respond to the out-of-the-ordinary stimuli and stress that are inherent in running.

What should you aim for in warm-up activities? Exercises that will contribute to your muscular and skeletal flexibility and,

Before And After The Run

to a lesser degree, strength. Also, you want exercises that will get your heart, blood, and lungs working at more than a casual or resting level.

One of the foremost guides to physical fitness, the *Official YMCA Physical Fitness Handbook,* emphasizes the importance of warm-ups and defines what they should include and how they should be carried out. The *YMCA Handbook* recommends exercises that: (1) Stretch muscles and joints to their full extent without straining; (2) are rhythmic in nature with one movement flowing naturally into the next; (3) combine muscle stretching with increased cardiovascular activity; (4) include all parts of the body; and (5) gradually increase in intensity as the warm-up progresses. In addition, there should be enough variety to make the warm-up interesting and enjoyable.

We subscribe to these thoughtful guidelines and urge you to do so as well. How you go about it is, of course, up to you. We caution you only to be sure that you do not overdo the warm-up or you will be taking away from your potential in the run. After all, the warm-up is simply a help to your running, just as running is a help to your physical fitness and general health. Overdoing either can have results exactly the opposite of those you are seeking.

There are all kinds of calisthenic exercises you can do to warm up for jogging. There are also various techniques for getting your circulatory and respiratory systems stimulated for the coming run. Select the ones that are the most comfortable and enjoyable for you. You must, however, know the parts of the body that are affected by a particular exercise. Don't just use the ones you remember from the days when you were training with the high-school basketball team or the nights you belonged to that physical fitness class some years ago. You can find information easily enough by consulting any book devoted to calisthenics, exercising, or physical fitness in general.

There are so many calisthenic exercises to choose from, we could not hope to present all of them here. Just loosely shaking your limbs (hands, arms, feet, and legs) and running in place are excellent warm-up efforts. Beyond these, we have selected ten warm-up activities designed to cover the most basic phases of conditioning. You will find them at the end of this chapter. These exercises will work on muscles and joints as well as preparing the heart and lungs. The sequence in which you do the exercises does not matter. And, we repeat, ten minutes is more than sufficient for the entire warm-up period.

Cooling Down

At the same track meet where all those runners and jumpers were warming up, you would have seen the distance racers cooling down after their run. They didn't simply stop, walk over, and pick up a medal if they won or amble off to the locker room if they lost. They knew from experience what to do, and they continued to run after the race was over — slower to be sure, but they were tapering off the running experience. Some runners bounce in place after the cooling-down run; others do some mild calisthenics — whatever suits their individual needs and preferences.

Stopping a vigorous run abruptly can be dangerous. Sudden relaxation after a demanding session of running can result in lightheadedness, dizziness, nausea, and even fainting. What we advise strongly is that you come out of your run gradually and smoothly. Let your body return to its normal state at a moderate rate. Remember, the blood has been going to your muscles, and now it is being diverted back to its normal circulation pattern and you do not want that shift to be too abrupt. Without a cooling off period, blood will pool in the feet and lower legs, depriving the brain of needed oxygen.

In addition, fatigue creates a build-up of lactic acid in the muscles. A cool-down helps dissipate the lactic acid and thus eases muscle aches and makes cramping less likely.

James Fixx, author and runner, advocates a relatively long cool-down: "Try to devote eight or ten minutes to cooling down in order to help work the metabolic wastes [such as lactic acid] out of your muscles. By the time you stop, your pulse should be within 20 beats of what it is when you aren't exercising." Dr.

Before And After The Run

Cooper suggests: "Five minutes of walking or very slow jogging eases the transition between running and resting."

Weather conditions, too, can have an effect when you bring your jogging to a halt. In cold weather, a sudden stop may bring on chills, for example, and make you more susceptible to colds, fever, and other ailments. And among the worst things you can do on either cold or warm days is to step immediately into a hot shower, a hot whirlpool bath, or sauna without adequately cooling down first.

The way you cool down is, like almost everything else in this book, a matter of personal preference. But some slow jogging, walking, or mild calisthenics as a cool-down should be an integral part of your running program.

What we are saying is simple. The running experience should be a three-part cycle: warm-up; run; cool-down. The first and last of the three do not need to be long, drawn-out affairs. They should be short and effective, and as natural as putting on and taking off your running shoes.

We urge you to remember that you are running for the sake of your fitness and your health; you want to contribute to those things, not detract from them. The best way to do that is to go about running in the best way possible, and that is by warming up before and cooling down after each run.

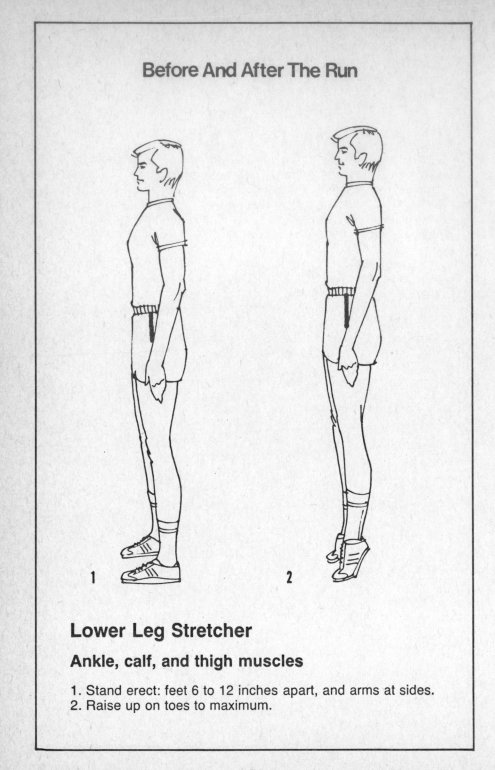

Lower Leg Stretcher

Ankle, calf, and thigh muscles

1. Stand erect: feet 6 to 12 inches apart, and arms at sides.
2. Raise up on toes to maximum.

Before And After The Run

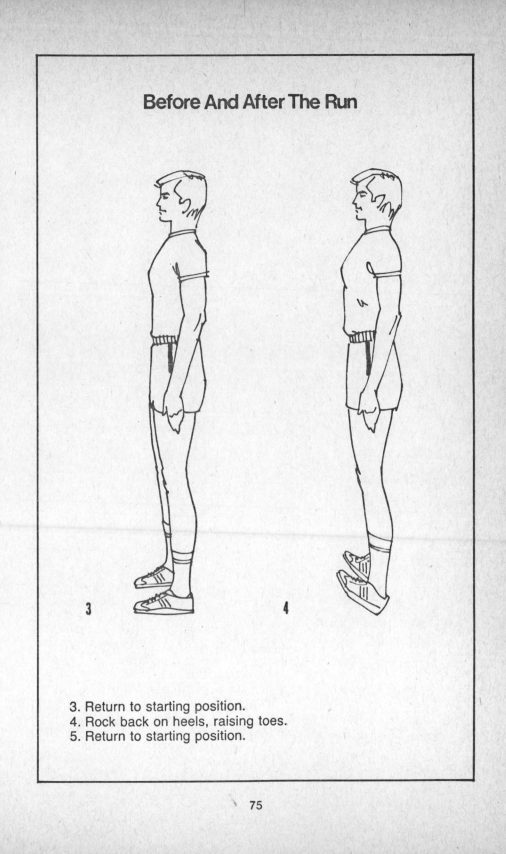

3

4

3. Return to starting position.
4. Rock back on heels, raising toes.
5. Return to starting position.

Before And After The Run

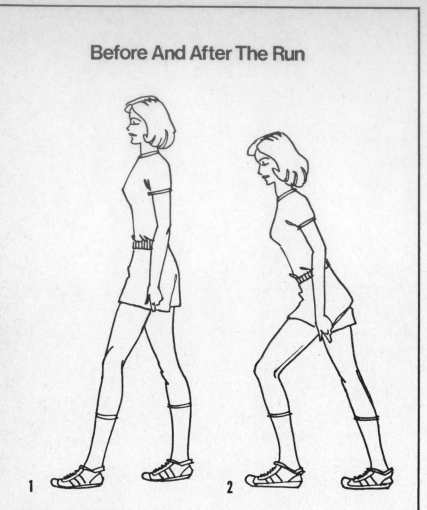

1   2

Step In Place

Achilles tendon, and calf and hamstring muscles

1. Stand erect: left foot directly in front of right foot with at least 12 inches separating left heel from right toes, and arms at sides.
2. Bend left knee forward, keeping right foot flat on the floor. You will feel tension in the muscles at the back of the right leg.
3. Return to starting position.
4. Repeat exercise with right foot forward and left foot back.

Before And After The Run

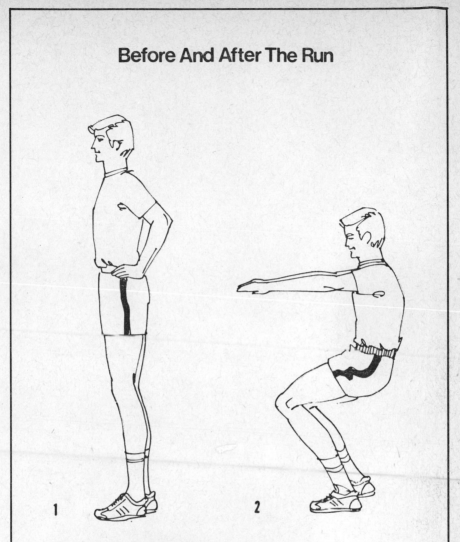

1

2

Modified Knee-Bends

Leg, thigh, and buttock muscles

1. Stand erect: shoulders squared, feet 6 to 12 inches apart, hands on hips or extended in front of body (whichever enables you to balance better).
2. Lower body by bending knees until you reach a half-squat position.
3. Return to starting position.

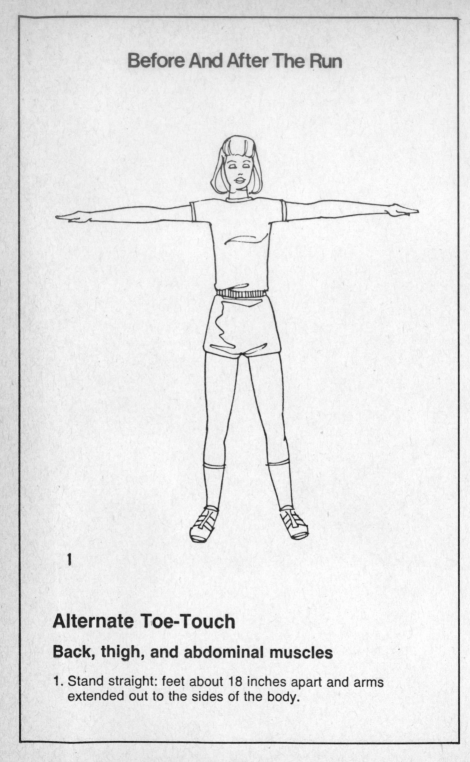

1

Alternate Toe-Touch

Back, thigh, and abdominal muscles

1. Stand straight: feet about 18 inches apart and arms extended out to the sides of the body.

Before And After The Run

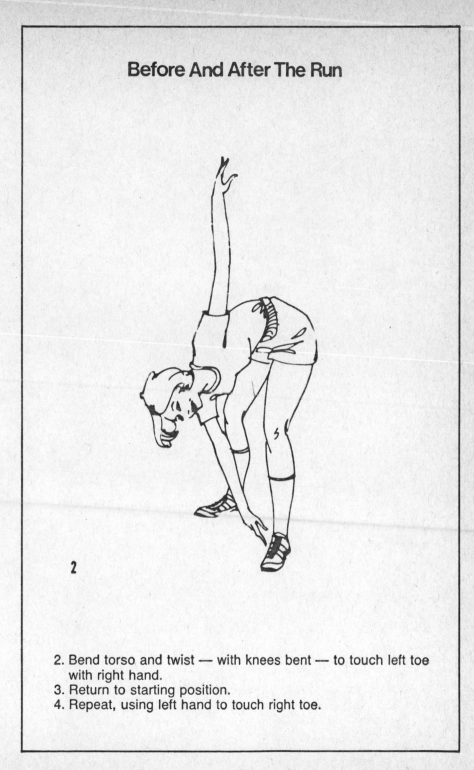

2

2. Bend torso and twist — with knees bent — to touch left toe with right hand.
3. Return to starting position.
4. Repeat, using left hand to touch right toe.

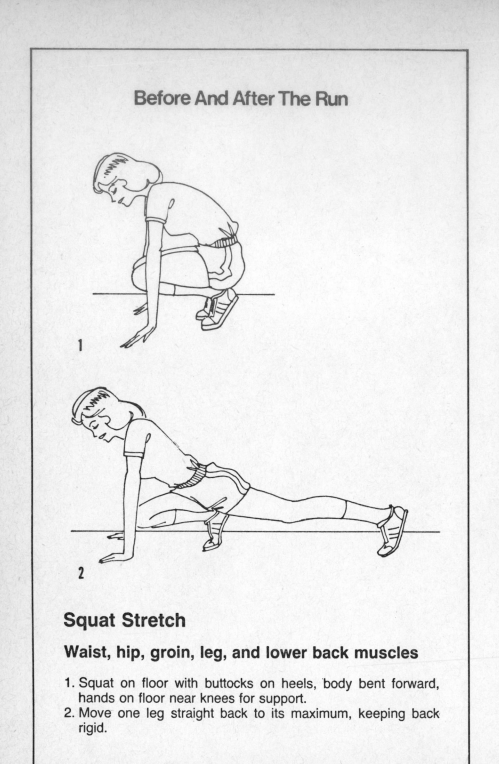

Squat Stretch

Waist, hip, groin, leg, and lower back muscles

1. Squat on floor with buttocks on heels, body bent forward, hands on floor near knees for support.
2. Move one leg straight back to its maximum, keeping back rigid.

Before And After The Run

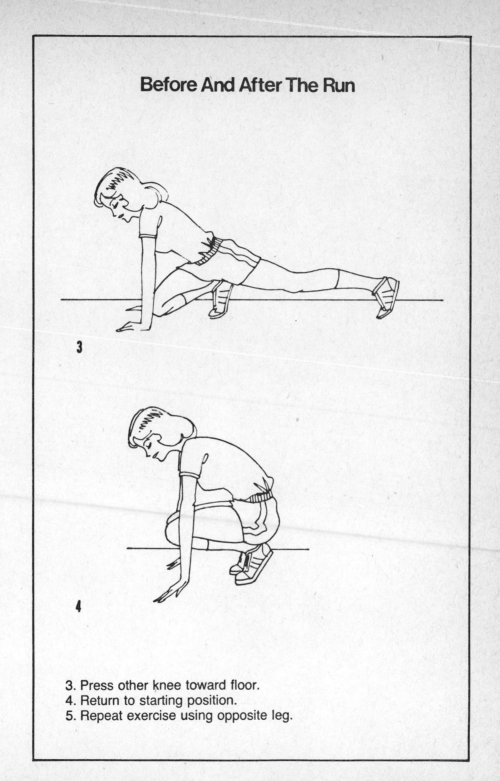

3

4

3. Press other knee toward floor.
4. Return to starting position.
5. Repeat exercise using opposite leg.

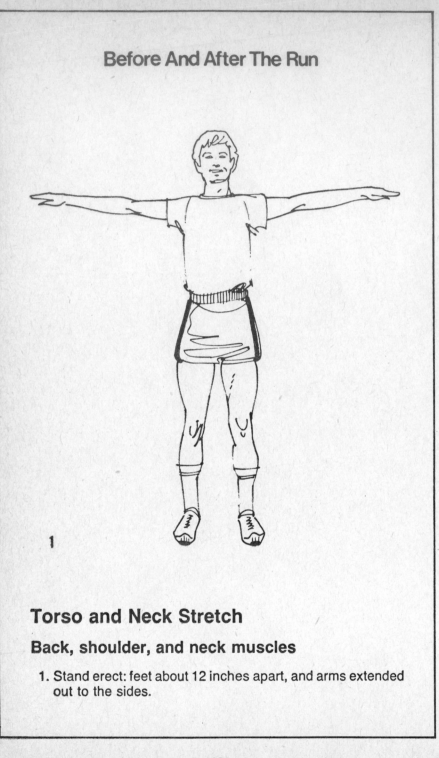

1

Torso and Neck Stretch

Back, shoulder, and neck muscles

1. Stand erect: feet about 12 inches apart, and arms extended out to the sides.

Before And After The Run

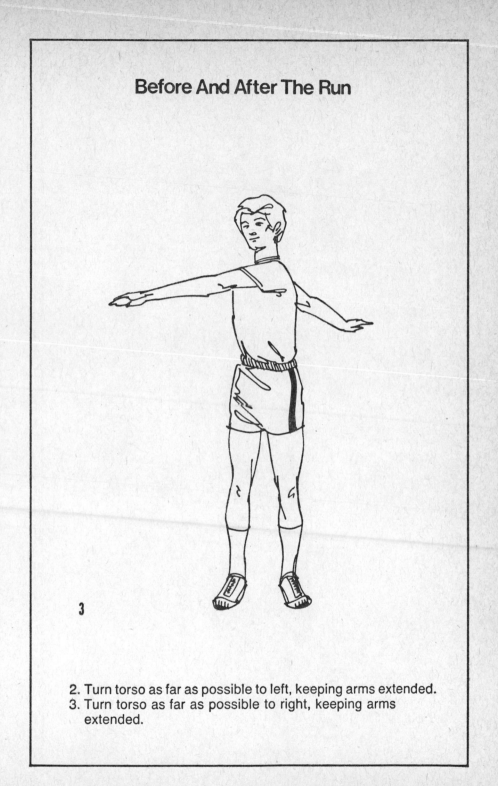

3

2. Turn torso as far as possible to left, keeping arms extended.
3. Turn torso as far as possible to right, keeping arms extended.

Before And After The Run

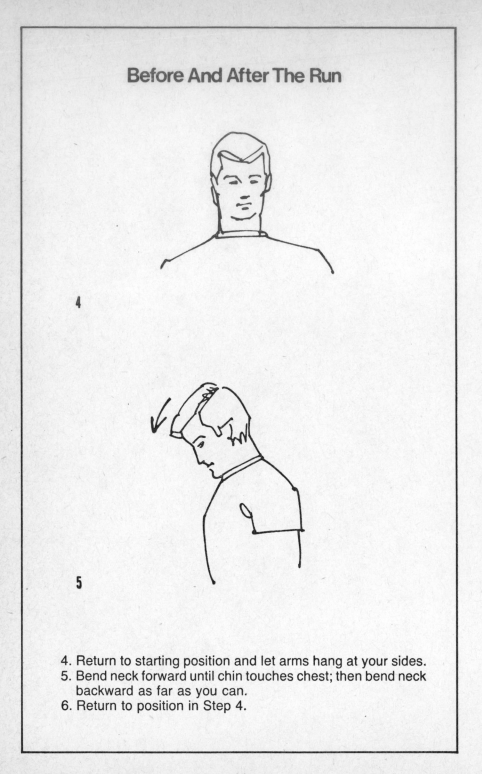

4

5

4. Return to starting position and let arms hang at your sides.
5. Bend neck forward until chin touches chest; then bend neck backward as far as you can.
6. Return to position in Step 4.

Before And After The Run

7

9

7. Turn head all the way to one side and then all the way to other side.
8. Return to position in Step 4.
9. Roll head in circular motion.
10. Return to position in Step 4.

Before And After The Run

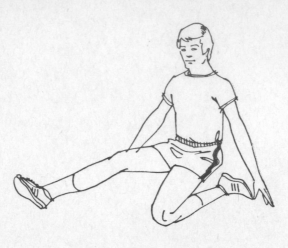

1

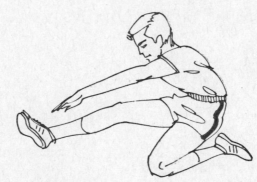

2

Hurdler's Stretch

Lower leg, thigh, abdominal, and back muscles

1. Sit on floor: right leg extended out in front and left leg bent at the knee and out to the side and hands at sides.
2. Reach out with left hand and touch toe of extended right foot.
3. Return hand to starting position.
4. Repeat several times.
5. Do complete exercise with left leg extended, using right hand to touch left toe.

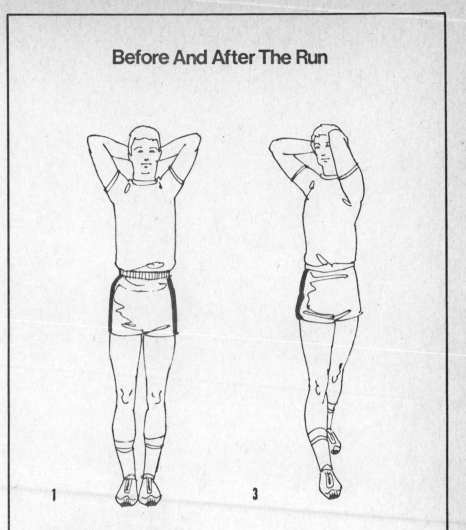

1   3

Walking Twist

Respiration, circulation, and back, abdominal, and groin muscles

1. Stand straight with hands clasped behind head.
2. Begin walking forward.
3. Twist body so opposite shoulder and elbow move in direction of lead foot.
4. As other foot comes forward, turn body so opposite elbow and shoulder rhythmically twist toward that foot.

Before And After The Run

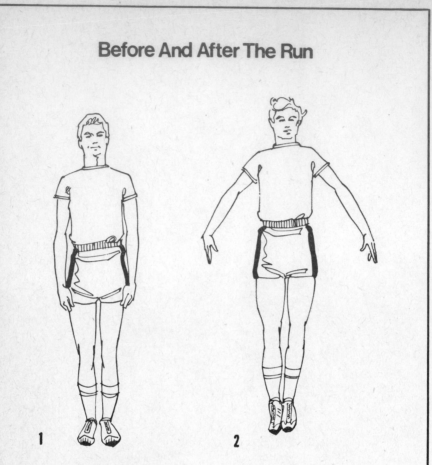

1   **2**

Jumping In Place

Respiration, circulation, and almost all muscle groups

1. Assume a relaxed standing position, arms hanging loosely at sides.
2. Jump with both feet, bouncing easily and slowly, with feet leaving the ground a few inches.
3. Gradually increase the speed and height of jump, while moving arms in a circular motion as if rope-skipping.
4. Switch to alternately bouncing on first one foot and then the other.
5. Reduce height and speed gradually and return to starting position.

Before And After The Run

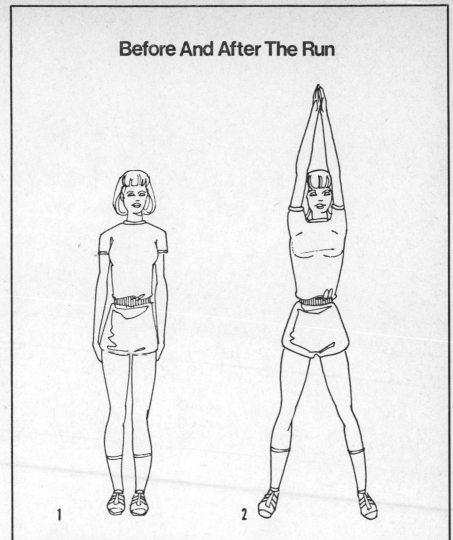

1 2

Side-Straddle-Hop

Respiration and leg and lower back muscles

1. Stand erect: feet together and arms at sides, with palms touching sides.
2. Jump into a straddle position, at the same time clapping hands above the head.
3. Jump back to starting position, lowering arms back to sides at the same time.

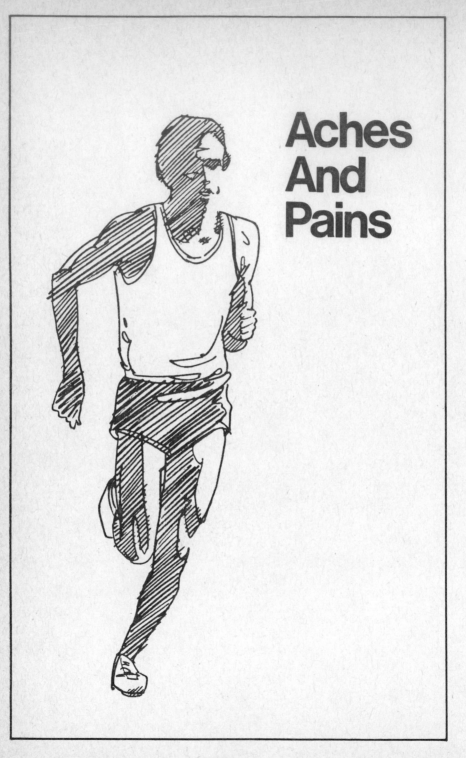

Aches
And
Pains

Aches And Pains

FRANK SHORTER, U.S. Olympic champion and one of the outstanding marathon runners of all time, spent the evening before the 1972 Olympic marathon drinking beer. As he explained it later, he was "trying to forget how much I'd suffer once I started to run." The list of physical ailments Shorter has suffered in the course of his running career might stretch as far as some of his runs.

Must you expect to suffer this way when you take up running? The answer, of course, is, "No," not if you simply want to make your life more interesting and improve your health by running. People like Shorter and other world class distance runners engage in a fierce kind of competition that inevitably punishes the body. Most of you, on the other hand, are unlikely to begin Olympic training or to try running a grueling 26-mile race in less than three hours.

Our goal is not to transform people who might be sitting too much or eating too much or breathing too hard into lithe and lean basket cases. It wouldn't make much sense to exchange one set of ailments for another. But you're kidding yourself if you think you can take your body from relative inertia to strenuous exercise without hearing it cry out "Stop, oh stop!" once in a while. So, in this chapter we'd like to prepare you for some of the new things you can expect to feel as your body gets used to running, and suggest ways for you to cope with them.

Coping With Pain

The experience of pain is strictly a private matter. Two people might be struck on the head with the same force by the same person using the same club, but each would feel it differently. Their nervous systems are not alike and neither are their cultural backgrounds or their experiences with pain.

Aches And Pains

So as you begin, and continue, to run, you will undoubtedly gather your own little private collection of twinges, throbs, aches, pains, and general distress that will lead you to discover "muscles you didn't even know you had," and "body noises" completely new to you. Dr. Kostrubala, for example, had his "click." He tells of hearing a strange clicking sound coming from somewhere during one of his runs. It wasn't until he assured himself that he was completely alone that he realized the sound was coming from his own neck. To this day he does not know what caused it or why it suddenly decided to appear. But he simply rotated his neck a few times and kept on running. Eventually the sound disappeared.

However unique or common your body noises and pains turn out to be, you are the best judge of what they mean. So pay attention to them. Draw on the experience of others whenever you can to understand your own afflictions. There are certain general guidelines for preventing or at least limiting your pain, and we'll be talking about that later in this chapter. But they may or may not work for you. Get together with other runners and ask them about pain they may be having and what they are doing about it. Try out things you think might work. If the pain persists, try something else.

Often the solution is simple enough, but finding it takes a little imagination and close observation of what you are doing. Dr. Sheehan, for example, found that one way to eliminate a continuing pain in his left knee was to switch the direction of his run. He had made a habit of running with the flow of traffic along the road. After putting up with the pain for a while he decided to try running against the flow of the traffic, and the pain went away. The cause was not psychological, nor the solution magical. It was simply the slant of the road that had gradually created an imbalance in his running style and a strain on his left knee. Had he been running on a banked indoor track, both the problem and the solution would have been the same.

Take comfort, then. Here you have Sheehan, an expert, working out problems of pain just like all the rest of us; "occupational hazards" shared by veteran and novice alike. Everyone will go through pain, more and less. It's nice to know you will not be alone when your turn comes. Most of the pain can be relieved.

Aches And Pains

Prevention

All along we have been stressing the value of running as a cardiovascular exercise designed not so much to tone up the muscles of the body as to strengthen the heart and lungs. When we run we simply use the skeleton and the muscles of the body to get the latter job done. The interesting thing about this is that those organs we mainly want to exercise — heart and lungs — are not the chief source of most of our pains but rather our feet, ankles, legs, and the rest of the body's apparatus that has to work so hard to exercise the heart and lungs.

Keeping to a minimum the amount of pain this running apparatus will suffer requires that you do three essential things: (1) Take good care of your feet; (2) strengthen the muscles, ligaments, tendons, and joints of the feet, legs, and back; and (3) develop flexibility in the body's muscular and skeletal systems.

It shouldn't be surprising that care of the feet heads the list. They take the most direct shocks as they propel you over all kinds of surfaces. These 52 oddly shaped bones kind of crunched together inside a couple of little skin bags are really rather wonderful.

They take the most punishment; so caring for them is the single most important thing a runner can do to prevent or alleviate distress. By trial and error and by talking to other runners, Dr. Sheehan discovered that improper care can cause pain in the knees and legs as well as the feet.

Take a look at your running shoes. With your socks they are the only protection your feet have as they continually beat against the running surface. Do they fit properly? Does your foot sort of squish around or rub against the inside, even a little, or is there too little room? Are they laced tightly enough, or do they cut off circulation?

Socks that are too thick diminish the blood's circulation if they make your feet, in effect, too large for the shoes you are using. Thin socks, on the other hand, cannot give your feet the cushions they need. Thick or thin, your socks should fit your foot nicely, so that they don't bunch up inside your shoe to create irritation and blisters.

Once the runner begins to feel little irritations in his feet, however minor they may be, he automatically reacts to them, and unconsciously favors this or that until he abandons his natural running style altogether. As a consequence, he introduces stresses that weren't there before and eventually generates pains elsewhere in his body.

Before the Run

Conditioning your muscles, ligaments, joints, and tendons is a process that will take place naturally and automatically as you run. But you can help it along by supplementing your running with calisthenics or other exercises geared to developing strength and flexibility. They do not benefit the heart and lungs, but they can prepare the body to gain more from an aerobic exercise like running. If your muscles and joints are conditioned to work under great stress with a minimum of pain, running will be a far greater joy for you than otherwise, in the beginning and for as long as you run.

If you set up a regular exercise program for yourself to parallel your running program, be sure it is broad and thorough enough to condition all the parts of your body. The legs, ankles, and feet are more directly involved in running than anything else. But you don't want to short-change the lower back, the upper torso, and the arms. Raising yourself on your toes, touching your toes, sit-ups, knee-bends, squat-thrusts, hurdler's stretches, and yoga limbering exercises all contribute to the conditioning of the muscular and skeletal systems.

The main thing to remember is that none of this is done for the sake of appearance. It may be that all these exercises will end up giving you a comely, even powerful, body — and perhaps the courage to kick sand in the face of that beach bully who used to pick on you when you were just a 98-pound weakling. But that's frosting on the cake. Muscular changes that help you run better and with less pain — that's what you will be working on.

If you do not want to get this serious about exercises, you should at least work a few into your jogging program. In a

Aches And Pains

preceding chapter we said that much of the pain you will feel when you start to jog can be diminished or even avoided if you warm up beforehand. Just a few stretching exercises should be enough to ease the body into more strenuous activity.

During The Run: A Question Of Style

Experienced athletes move with grace and economy of motion. Most of us, however, have to learn the right way to run. An improper running style can cause unnecessary strain and lead to injuries.

Don't land on your heels or your toes. Dr. Cooper's advice is to run flat-footed. Touch down on the flat of your foot, then roll your weight forward from heel to toe. He further recommends that you keep your knees flexed, so that the impact of the foot striking the ground will be partly absorbed, much like the action of a shock absorber on your car.

Lean slightly forward so that your weight is over your front foot. Keep your stride fairly short and your arms bent at about a 90-degree angle. Your arms should be close to the body, moving just ahead of and behind your torso as you run. Don't clench your hands into fists — this makes your muscles tense. Remind yourself to relax your jaw, shoulders, and hands as often as necessary.

After the Run

When your run is over and your cool-down completed, treat yourself to a long soak in a hot tub. It will help relieve any soreness or pain you may have. If it does nothing else, a hot bath should relax you thoroughly. A whirlpool bath is best, since it combines a kind of massaging action with heat. But they aren't very common or accessible to most people, so just hop in your own tub at home.

For severe localized pain, try ice, a time-honored pain reliever. Just freeze water ahead of time in rigid plastic cups so it is easy to handle when you want to use it. Then, when you get back from your run and some of your muscles are crying "uncle," all you have to do is take a cup out of the freezer and rub it back and forth over the painful spot. The coldness of the ice pack will cause your blood vessels to constrict. When they dilate again the blood will carry off toxins from the affected area. At the same time, the increased circulation will carry whatever nutrients or protective organisms the body needs to repair the inflamed tissues.

Normal Complaints, Aches, And Pains

Anybody who takes up running seriously, or even casually, will have to endure one or more of the aches and pains we'll be talking about. The most superbly conditioned runner may not be entirely free of them. So let's start "from the ground up."

The Toes

Most of the distress felt in the toes comes from poorly fitted running shoes. Charles Kuntzleman, consultant to the YMCA on physical fitness, offers this advice: "When you are trying on a new pair of running shoes, be sure they fit well at the toe section. Shoe widths are measured across the widest part of the foot sole, and sometimes tend to taper too drastically in the toe area." Other brands, he adds, "may be too wide there for your particular foot. Be sure the fit is right for *you*." It is quite true that the size of a running shoe gives no real indication of the fit you can expect for your foot. The shape of your foot finally determines the shoe you should choose for maximum comfort. So select a design that matches your foot as closely as possible (see "Rating The Running Shoes" for some helpful suggestions).

Few things are more aggravating to a runner than toenails that cut into the flesh of the toes every time his foot comes down against the ground. The solution is as simple as the problem is painful: keep your toenails trimmed, especially at the corners.

Aches And Pains

In the foot's longest bones, the metatarsals, the stress of running can produce fractures so small they may not even be visible on an X-ray. Normally they will not have to be splinted or put into a cast. They simply heal all by themselves. But it takes time, maybe a month or two, even if you do not subject them to severe strain. This doesn't mean you have to interrupt your running program while they heal. But during this time it would be wise to run on very soft surfaces at a reduced pace and for shorter distances.

Blisters

If you detect even a slight friction or tickling sensation in any part of your foot, you may be feeling the onset of a blister. To keep it from growing worse, apply a liberal coat of Vaseline to the area. But if the Vaseline is used too late and you come home sporting a full-fledged blister, treat it right away. It can become infected. Wash the foot thoroughly and apply an antiseptic to the blister and the tissue around it. Then tape it over with gauze.

Jogger's Heel

This term is reserved for a group of heel problems that include bone bruises and heel spurs — painful bony growths on the heel bone itself. These ailments are normally caused by running on a hard surface, stepping on sharp objects with force enough to cause a bruise, or wearing poorly designed running shoes. These complaints don't lend themselves to a quick cure. Rest is good for them, but not always desirable for the person who wants to maintain his or her conditioning. Heel "donuts" or heel cups, designed to be worn inside the shoe to ease the pain, are available in most sporting goods stores or mail-order houses that cater to runners.

The Achilles Tendon

The Achilles tendon is the thick tendon at the back of the leg that connects the heel and foot to the back of the calf muscles.

Aches And Pains

It controls the hinge-like action of the ankle with every running step and therefore does a lot of work during a run. Tendinitis is not produced by sudden stress as in a sprain, but by the excessive use of a tendon during vigorous exercise. Achilles tendinitis is a very painful condition and not easy to get rid of.

Tendons frequently become inflamed and swollen when they are constricted by equipment. If you feel pain in your Achilles tendons your running shoes could be the culprit. The heels may be too low or too hard, or the back seam too tight, putting a strain on the tendon or crowding it. Perhaps the arch support in the shoe is not adequate.

Achilles tendinitis can also be caused by years of wearing heeled shoes. The heels favored by Americans shorten the Achilles tendons and makes them less resilient. The very act of running often tightens these tendons even more, just as it develops the muscles of the legs. This is one reason that stretching exercises are so important to the runner. They limber up the tendons and counteract the effects of running and wearing heels.

Stretching calisthenics can be useful, but more and more runners are using yoga exercises. Yoga is a system of exercise that stretches and limbers the muscles and joints, adding greatly to flexibility.

Shin Splints

Anyone who is not used to running will probably suffer from shin splints at some point. Shin splints create sensations of extreme tenderness and pain running down the front of the leg from the knee to the ankle. It is a common ailment, principally caused by the shin muscles pulling at the membranes surrounding them and at the shinbone to which they are attached. According to most authorities, shin splints will show up sooner if you run on hard surfaces. Therefore, if you have been running on cement or anything like it, switch to a gentler surface like grass. And check your shoes. Sometimes low-heeled running shoes can bring relief. Stretching exercises, particularly those that stretch the hamstring and the Achilles tendon, are very helpful. Designed mainly to benefit the back of the legs, they are surprisingly effective in curing shin splints.

Aches And Pains

Jogger's Knee

The human knee can stand a remarkable degree of stress and still work pretty well. That it is able to survive even one brutal crush by several 250-pound professional football players hitting it from different angles, strains our belief. But that happens, thousands of times, every winter weekend. Fortunately, runners like us do not have to sacrifice our knees for the glory of pro football. Still, on your anonymous run through the neighborhood or along the beach, your knees are not completely safe from stress. Usually, pains are associated with the kneecap, beneath it or along its sides. Sometimes the kneecap does not articulate smoothly against the lower end of the thighbone as it should, and the knee becomes increasingly irritated and swollen as you run. If you have this problem, you may have to curtail your running program. But first, experiment with different running methods, because a lot of doctors think that this problem may be caused — or if not caused, then aggravated — by the way your foot strikes the ground.

Dr. Sheehan's knee problem, mentioned earlier, was not caused by his stride so much as by the sloping road. In compensating for that he introduced unnatural stresses into his knee action and created his knee problem. If you run indoors on a banked track in one direction for long distances, say 20 to 25 laps, your ankles as well as your knees will be subject to these same unnatural stresses.

Cramps and Spasms

A cramp can suddenly seize any muscle and be exceedingly painful. It is an involuntary contraction of the muscle, but so far nobody has explained the cause of cramps to everybody's satisfaction. You can get a cramp without exercising at all — during sleep, for example. But as a general rule, cramps give us fits during prolonged exercise. Runners are much more likely to suffer from cramps and spasms in the muscles of the calf and in the feet than non-runners.

When you first take up running your muscles may tend to cramp up or go into spasms rather frequently. Dr. Sheehan

recommends about 30 minutes of swimming a day as an anti-
dote until they simply go away. Both Bill Bowerman and James
Fixx suggest you add a little salt to your diet. In most cases, as
you continue to run and your muscular condition improves, you
should be troubled less and less with the complaint. But count
yourself among the lucky if spasms and cramps disappear altogether.

Sprains

While cramps and spasms are essentially painful contractions
of muscle tissue, a sprain is a rupture. When a sprain occurs, a
ligament, tendon, or even a muscle tears with a sudden twist or
movement that is more than the tissue can support. Small blood
vessels in the area break, and pain develops when the surrounding tissue swells up and overstimulates sensitive nerve
endings.

Because the ankle becomes such a vulnerable pivot when
you are running, ankle twists and sprains are fairly common.
Obviously you should watch where you are going. This means
that, even if you are the casual type and not too finicky about
running on any kind of ground, you should at least learn how to
pick your way among the potholes and skillfully sidestep any
beer cans that may be littering your path.

If you aren't very good at that and manage to sprain an ankle,
you will have to postpone further running until it is healed.

Side Stitch

The side stitch, like shin splints, is a common affliction among
runners, especially beginners, who run too hard and too fast
before they are in good enough condition. The pain is sharp
and usually makes itself felt just under the rib cage. The side
stitch is thought to be the cramping of a muscle in the abdomi-
nal region, perhaps the diaphragm muscle.

Dr. Kostrubala says that the best thing you can do when a
side stitch strikes is to concentrate on it and keep on running. It
is nothing to worry about and will eventually disappear. You
might also try changing your stride momentarily, blowing all the

air out of your lungs in one burst, yelling as loud as you can, or singing a song at the top of your voice — whatever pleases you. Or, if you want to attract much less attention from onlookers, just limit yourself to breathing deeply. If none of these work and you can't get rid of the stitch, you can learn to live with it. Fortunately, this is rarely necessary.

Serious Aches And Pains

The pains we have been talking about up to now are what we might call "routine" complaints. Most runners have them, recognize them for what they are, try to do what they can about them, and then ignore them. If you pamper yourself and worry over every little twinge as you start creaking into shape, you probably never will become a runner.

But the symptoms described in this section are signals you should *always* heed. They are important warnings your body gives out to tell you to go no farther. When you get them, bring your running to a halt, remembering to cool down if possible.

Back Pains

Back pains should not be fooled around with, particularly if they occur in the lower back, the result, perhaps, of a slipped spinal disc. Obviously, back problems cannot be diagnosed on the running path, but if you have a slipped disc, you'll know it, and fast.

Some lower back pains result from exercising after years of relative inactivity. You will have to guess at the seriousness of these pains by the way you feel at the time; that is, how intense they are, how much they cripple you, and so on. In any case, go slow. Feel your way. If for any reason you think further exercise might cause any harm, discontinue running and consult your physician about the pain.

If the problem does not seem to be serious, causing only

minor discomfort, and does not increase as you continue to run, Dr. Cooper suggests that you supplement your running exercise with a few calisthenics to strengthen your lower back, say 15 to 20 push-ups and the same number of sit-ups with your knees bent.

Quite a few runners have found that their back pains disappeared after this kind of double exercise program. But we're not promoting any miracle cures. On the contrary, we urge you to be extremely cautious. If you have back trouble and do not approach running with common sense and care, you can make the condition worse.

Dizziness

Dizziness is another warning sign you should respond to without hesitation. It can indicate the early stages of heat exhaustion or heat stroke, especially if you are running in hot weather and the humidity is high. Even if it is neither hot nor humid, there can still be cause for alarm. Dizziness, particularly when it is accompanied by severe shortness of breath, can signify the presence of circulatory difficulties or other problems of major medical significance.

If you get any of these signals, stop until they go away, then begin again to jog very slowly. In most cases the experience will be momentary, no cause for worry, and disappear as quickly as it came. But if it recurs as you continue to exercise, stop running altogether and see your doctor.

Heart Problems

Be particularly wary of extreme and/or persistent pains in the arms, chest, neck, head, ears, or upper abdomen. Dr. Kostrubala cites the case of an internist who, curiously, suffered with such pains for an entire day before he gave in to them and decided he'd better get help. It was a heart attack, to no one's surprise but his, but he was lucky enough to survive.

If you experience any of these pains, we strongly suggest that you not be as hard-headed as he was. The symptoms of an attack can take different forms: a very heavy pressure, as if

Aches And Pains

someone were sitting on top of your chest; an extreme tightness inside the center of your chest, like a clenched fist; a feeling something like indigestion; a stuffiness high in your stomach or low in your throat. Whenever you have a strong symptom that even closely resembles any one of these, stop running at once and get to a physician.

You may have gone through a stress ECG before you started a running program and passed it with flying colors. If so, your chance of having this experience is relatively small. But don't get cocky. *Your* body, not somebody else's electronic measurements, has the final word. So listen to it.

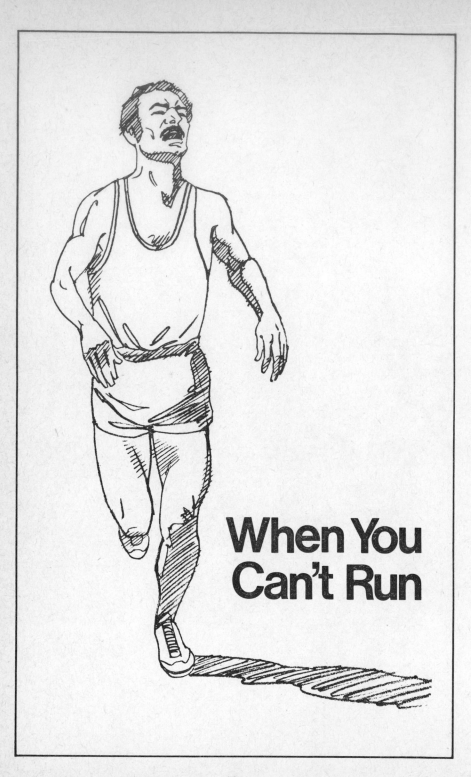

When You Can't Run

When You Can't Run

THE MOTTO of the U. S. Postal Service reads: "Neither snow, nor rain, nor heat, nor gloom of night stays these couriers from the swift completion of their appointed rounds."

Whether these words still describe mail carriers and the organization they work for is perhaps open to question. Dedicated runners, however, take this sentiment very much to heart. When asked what they do when running is impossible, many answered, "Cry." Though spoken with tongue in cheek, this plaintive response indicates the intensity of their commitment.

The beginner, on the contrary, may be tempted to heave a sigh of relief when the elements make running difficult. When the rain comes down in buckets, the sun is hot enough to dismay a camel, or the temperature low enough to delight a polar bear, it is all too easy to curl up with a good book, feeling virtuous because the weather and not the runner can take the blame.

The serious runner isn't so easily discouraged. Maintaining the physical fitness he or she has worked hard for is too important. Many runners derive great pleasure from jogging over fresh clean snow or through a hard rain. On days when running really isn't a good idea, they find alternative exercises. There are games to play and activities to engage in that are adequate short-term substitutes.

You do have to be selective, however. Many of the sports that people take up "for exercise" don't provide the cardiovascular exertion you need for fitness. Golf and bowling, for example, make almost no demands on the cardiovascular system. Even football, a far more vigorous game, consists of brief periods of violent play followed by longer rests or huddles. The exercise they offer is not sustained enough to contribute to cardiovascular fitness. There are a few games that are exceptions. Handball played by two excellent players, basketball, and volleyball can all be good sustained exercise.

On the whole, individual outdoor and gym activities are preferable for two reasons: You will not be dependent on the skills of another person and you will not be subject to the stop-and-start pattern found in most organized sports.

The exercise — or exercises — you choose as an alternative to running will depend on a number of things: where you live, the climate, geography, and topography, the availability of facilities, and, of course, your preferences. If you want to swim you need a pool. If you want to try handball, racquetball, or squash you need a court. If you want to ski and you live in Florida, you'll have to give up the idea or take a long trip.

There are, however, enough choices here for most people and most situations. And that's important. Dr. George Sheehan, veteran runner and spokesman for the sport, says that, "One man's play can, of course, be another man's boredom." We agree, and suggest the same is true for women. So pick one you know you like or at least think you might enjoy. That way you can use your alternative as often as necessary without sacrificing either conditioning or pleasure. You may even decide to break up your regular running program with other exercises to keep your interest level high.

Walking

This may seem like an unlikely alternative to jogging, but it can be an excellent one. You may be looking for an alternative because your feet and legs are not in condition to handle the shock of striking the pavement at high speed. Walking, however, may take enough of the strain off to let you continue exercising without aggravating the injury. Your feet will not be hitting the ground with anything like the force used in running.

It may be difficult to keep up your heart rate by simple walking alone, especially if you are in good condition. If you are in poor or mediocre shape, however, like most of us, walking may just be the exercise you need when running is too painful or otherwise impractical.

And, even for those of you in respectable condition, walking at high speed — "race walking," as some call it — may be the answer. As Dr. Sheehan points out: "The race walker . . . can make do with ordinary feet. He can put miles and miles and miles on feet that would break down in any other sport . . . Race walking is a safe refuge for any injured athlete."

Whatever your walking speed, it must keep your heart rate

within its target range for the required period of time — a minimum of 15 minutes — to be useful. You might want to spice up the effort with strenuous walking over difficult terrain, up steep grades, up and down stairs, and so forth.

Remember, walking, even race walking, is only a temporary measure. It will not be as much fun as running, now that you've gotten the hang of jogging but it is a handy way to work out without having to go to a gym, chase after a piece of exercise equipment, or find an open swimming pool. It is the most accessible alternative of all, and it can work for you whenever you feel you need to use it.

Running In Place

Your great enemy in this particular alternative will be boredom. Somehow the excitement of pounding away at the same few inches of real estate is less than breathtaking. To gaze dumbly for 15 minutes or more at the same patch of wall in your den is enough to put even your teeth to sleep. Living room joggers have tried all kinds of things to liven things up a bit — some watch television; others listen to music. Then there's always daydreaming. Nonetheless, running in place can be boring, boring, boring.

What running in place has going for it is the simple and inviting prospect of staying inside where it's warm while the wind howls along your favorite path. Having decided to pay the price of boredom to gain that comfort, you might have to pay another. For stationary running that's worth the effort, you will have to run vigorously. That means your feet should leave the floor a minimum of six inches and your tempo should be relatively fast. You will need to maintain your stationary running for periods of time equivalent to the level of your regular running program.

Since you have to lift your feet high without having the advantage of moving forward, running in place tends to put a great deal of stress on your feet and ankles. This happens even though it may not seem that you are exerting yourself as much as you really are. Dr. Cooper, in his book *The New Aerobics,* advises: "To avoid foot and ankle trouble, wear cushion-soled shoes and run on a soft surface, preferably on a thick rug." To that advice we might add our own, not related to the condition of your body but to the condition of your carpeting: If you are going to run in place, change the place from time to time. Otherwise you will end up with a shallow pit in the middle of your rug. If you happen to have a special attachment to your spot, however, get a piece of carpet about one foot square and use it.

We have never heard of anyone giving up their running, swimming, or bicycling programs to concentrate on running in place. But we have discovered quite a few serious joggers who use it as a substitute when they cannot get out into the streets. If you do it properly, the boredom will be worth it.

Cycling
In Place

Most of us have seen a curious contraption consisting of a frame, a seat, pedals, and a wheel. It rather resembles a bicycle that somebody forgot to finish. You plant yourself on the seat, pedal like crazy, and go nowhere. Some call it an exercycle and others an ergometer. We'll call it a stationary cycle. You can call it whatever you want. Whatever its name, and despite its strange appearance, it can keep you in shape while the rain comes down or a wrenched back heals.

Cycling in place is only a little less humdrum than running in place, but a lot more welcome to anybody living in the apartment below. But less boring is still boring, and stationary cyclists have had to resort to the same diversions as those who run in place in order not to drift into a state of mental numbness.

As you might expect, stationary cycles come in different models. Some are motorized, while you provide the power for others. On the motorized version, the pedals are turned by the motor which causes the seat to move and the handlebars to move forward and backward. The main purpose of all this is to

When You Can't Run

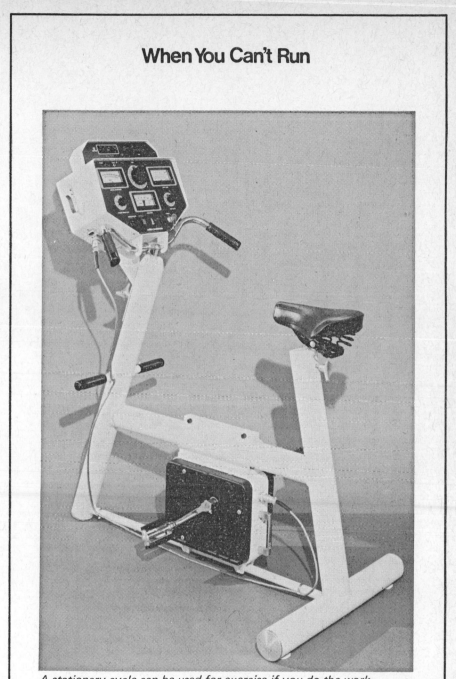

A stationary cycle can be used for exercise if you do the work yourself.

put the body into motion. There is a lot of movement, but very little real exertion, and consequently very little conditioning. It is possible, if you "work against" the motorized machine, to gain some beneficial cardiovascular exercise, but a lot more can be accomplished with the non-motorized version.

Certain features, such as speedometers and mileage indicators, can give the cyclist various goals to help sustain his or her interest. If you choose, you can set speed and distance goals and see if you can meet them. Most bikes that you pump include a knob that, when turned, increases the pedal resistance, duplicating, in effect, the gravity you must work against when you pump a normal bicycle up a hill.

These devices can help you adapt your cycling to the graduated schedule of your regular running program, longer distances, better times, and so on. The range of pedal resistance is great enough to tax even the most experienced runner, allowing him to stay within his heart rate range.

A good stationary cycle can cost more than a good bicycle. Prices range from about $75 for a basic machine with no features to several hundred dollars. If you do not want to spend that kind of money, you can often find stationary cycles at your local YMCA or YWCA, health clubs, or in some school and community gymnasiums.

Bicycling

This exercise presumes that you own a bike or can conveniently borrow or rent one. By its very nature it too can bring you excellent cardiovascular benefits. And it's possible to end up with a bonus or two. Since you can cover a lot of ground on a bike, you can use your ride for more than exercising your body. It can take you to school, to work, or on errands around town, while the car stays shut up in the garage or at the curb. When you get back home you can pat yourself on the back for having saved money on gasoline, helped solve the energy crisis in a small way, and given yourself a good workout, all at the same time.

When You Can't Run

That "good workout," however, depends on several things. First of all, to really help your heart and lungs you have to pedal hard enough to get your heart rate up into your heart range and keep it there.

For another, you'll have to fight "technological progress" every inch of the way. The Official YMCA Physical Fitness program makes an interesting observation about the modern bicycle and its use as a device for keeping and staying fit: ". . . employing road cycling for a controlled exercise program presents difficulties because there are many different kinds of bicycles and all kinds of roads. The invention of the 3-speed and then the 10-speed bike created the bicycle boom of recent years by enabling the rider to pedal up grades without dismounting." In short, technology has succeeded in shifting most of the work from your body to all those fancy gears, permitting you to make it up those steep grades without batting an eyelash. And, as it happens, without making your heart and lungs work. A little more technology like this and you might as well strap a side-car to your bike and hire a chauffeur to do the pedaling. Or, just take the car after all.

Of course, the simplest way to combat these "conveniences" is to demand that the gears give you back at least a little of the work. Forget you have about three-fourths of those chrome-plated gears. Let that giant sprocket serve as decoration while the sweat gleams on your brow. If there are hills around, don't avoid them. Look for areas that will let you ride for long distances without stopping, such as bicycle paths and country roads, away from traffic lights, automobiles, and pedestrians that force you to stop or let up on your exercise. The harder you have to pump and the fewer the interruptions, the better the physical conditioning you will get from it.

Swimming

The great thing about swimming is that it is one of the most enjoyable sports of all. It is not only one of the best overall

When You Can't Run

conditioning activities, but, like running, is a cardiovascular exercise of great value.

All the major fitness programs praise it for this reason. It is a main ingredient of Dr. Cooper's aerobics program. It is prescribed in large doses by the Official YMCA Physical Fitness program. It is highly recommended by the President's Council on Physical Fitness and Sports. It enjoys this reputation as one of the best alternatives to running — indeed, as a superb exercise in its own right — because it enables you to reach your target heart range easily and to maintain it for an extended period of time.

To use this as an alternative, you obviously need to know how to swim. But you don't have to be particularly good at it — just good enough to keep from sinking to the bottom of the pool. Even if you don't live near a large body of water you shouldn't have too much trouble finding a pool. They are pretty common. But the accessibility of a place to do your swimming is clearly something you have to take into account.

To get the maximum benefit from swimming, simply treat it as a running program. Swim for time, not speed or distance. But *swim;* don't just float around with your toes pointing in the air. Arrange your swimming program in graduated increments of time. A minimum of 15 continuous minutes of swimming is necessary to realize cardiovascular benefits.

It does not matter how you swim during those minutes; the Australian crawl, backstroke, sidestroke, breaststroke, butterfly, even the dog-paddle are fine as long as they keep your head above water, your body moving, and your heart rate up to your target range for at least 15 minutes or more.

Running is a demanding exercise. So is swimming. Approach it with the same caution we have advised in our running program and don't let your enthusiasm exceed your good sense. Begin slowly and build up gradually. You may be in relatively good condition from running, but you must remember that swimming requires you to use muscles that were only moderately employed in running, such as the muscles of the upper body and the lower back.

In swimming you probably have the finest alternative to running you can choose.

Rope Skipping

Leon Spinks and Sylvester Stallone do it very well. So do most little girls. But rope skipping is no longer restricted only to prize fighters and children. Rope skipping has been discovered to be an excellent form of cardiovascular exercise, easy to do with a little practice, and requiring very little in the way of equipment — a simple jump rope, available at just about any toy or sporting goods store.

How you do it is a matter of personal preference. As an interesting exercise rope skipping might at first appear to rank at about the same level as running in place. Actually, it can be kind of fun, at least for a while. Here at least, you can do something besides stare at the pattern of the living room drapes. You've got a rope to play with and you can do all sorts of things with your feet. Dr. Cooper suggests four different ways of skipping — there are undoubtedly many others for you to discover on your own, but these are certainly the basic ones: (1) Jump with both feet together. (2) Alternate left and right feet. (3) Jump up and down on one leg only. (4) Step over the rope one foot at a time, almost as if you were walking. You can have fun with these or any complicated patterns or combinations you can dream up, just so long as you keep going for the required period of time. And as long as you don't hang yourself.

We should warn you that it's quite impossible to skip for the required time in one continuous stretch. It may surprise you to learn that most people, even those in good condition, cannot skip without pausing after a few minutes because it is so demanding. So it is usually combined with other indoor exercises, such as running in place, or stationary cycling. The important thing is that you perform the combination of exercises at a level strenuous enough to maintain your target heart rate.

Besides being an extremely efficient exercise for cardiovascular training, rope skipping strengthens the muscles of the arms, shoulders, back, and legs, while developing your balance and physical coordination.

Treadmill Running Or Walking

The equipment, — a treadmill, obviously — required for this exercise comes in motorized and non-motorized models like the stationary cycle. But here the relative value of the two designs is reversed: the motorized version of the treadmill is the better of the two for exercise purposes.

Running on a motorized treadmill is as close to real running as you can get without actually hitting the street. You simulate the run almost exactly. Many motorized treadmills can be inclined to imitate walking or running uphill, making the exercise more difficult and improving its value.

Non-motorized treadmills, driven by your own muscle power, are uncomfortable and difficult to sustain for long periods of time. Ranging in price from $100 to $300, they are considerably less expensive than motorized treadmills, which can cost between $500 and $2500, with most of them priced at over $1000.

You still face the problem of boredom. You always will in a situation where you work hard without going anywhere. But at least you are duplicating the run almost exactly and getting the most out of your effort.

Rowing Machines

This is another one of those exercises that can be a good alternative according to experts, who say it not only exercises the heart and lungs, but most of the body. The rowing can become quite strenuous, since you can adjust the rowing tension higher and higher. It makes severe demands on the muscular system, since it forces you to use most of the major muscle groups in both the lower and upper body. The arms and legs pull and extend, the back is stretched as you lean forward to

When You Can't Run

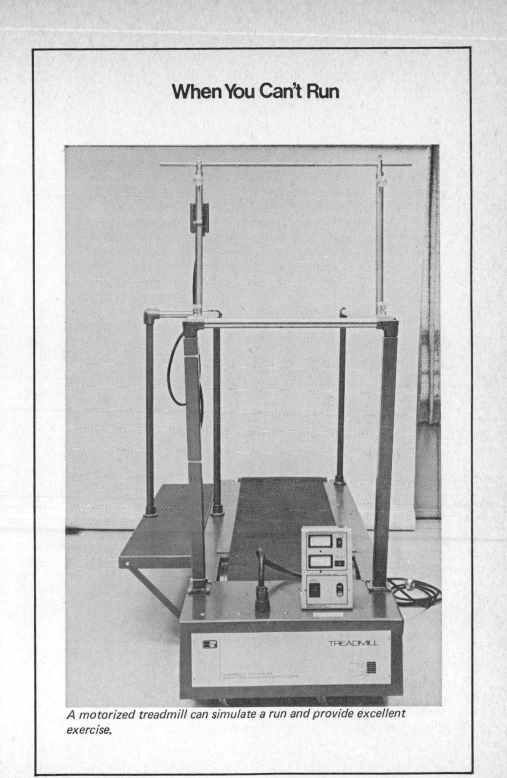

A motorized treadmill can simulate a run and provide excellent exercise.

begin a new stroke, and its major muscles are brought into play by pulling the oars back. In fact, fitness experts suggest that the demands made on these muscle groups limit, to some degree at least, the amount of cardiovascular conditioning possible in this exercise. The exercise itself is strenuous enough to force the heart to beat within its target range, but the muscles of the body work so hard in rowing that the average person finds it difficult to sustain the exercise long enough to really give the heart and lungs an extended workout. For this reason rowing might be best used, like rope skipping, in conjunction with another cardiovascular exercise that sustains the target rate without tiring the muscular system. Then the two exercises could be done one after the other and give the heart and lungs a workout that brings real benefits.

The rowing machine is not recommended for use by people with high blood pressure or victims of heart disease.

Cross-Country Skiing

This is one of the few alternate exercises for which adverse weather conditions are, in a sense, needed. Cross-country skiing is truly invigorating for every part of the body. You will use nearly all your muscles and improve your balance and coordination as well. But its most important benefit lies in its excellence as a cardiovascular exercise, equal to serious running and swimming, which is about as good as you can get.

It does require knowledge and skill to do this exercise. People have broken their legs and ankles in cross-country skiing, just as they have in downhill skiing. While you've got to know what you are doing, learning it will not take a whole series of costly lessons. Basic books on the subject should be sufficient, along with a little cautious practice. Lessons are available, if you feel you need them, at ski resorts and in many towns and cities across the snowbelt.

When You Can't Run

Most of these towns and cities are beginning to allocate areas specifically for cross-country skiing, since interest in the sport is on the rise. So, even for the city dweller, finding a place for this exercise is becoming less and less of a problem. If, however, there is no such area near you, remember that there is perhaps no more pleasant outing than to pack up your cross-country skis and head out to the country, a forest preserve, or a large park for a good workout.

Handball, Racquetball, And Squash

These three sports are treated together because they generate basically the same degree of exercise. But whether they qualify as true cardiovascular alternatives to running depends upon how vigorously they are played.

Their inherent game pattern is "start-stop": An opponent serves for a point, a point is made, one pattern is completed, and another begins. So the value of the three exercises depends entirely upon the skill of the players and the speed of the game.

In any case, as games, they are as strenuous as any in sport, and ideally require a nearly constant activity which can keep the heart pumping and the lungs gasping for fresh quantities of oxygen.

Keep in mind that these games require you to be in good condition. They are not alternatives for the exerciser who has just recently moved from a sedentary lifestyle into elementary physical activity. You will be taxing yourself to the limit in these sports, and to do that you must be in condition.

We offer this tip: play these sports with someone who plays at your level. This makes for a better game and keeps the exercise going with fewer periods of rest and fewer stops.

Be sure to warm up and cool down properly if you plan to participate in these sports. Don't jump into a hot shower as soon as you are through, and don't just walk in off the street and into a spirited game. Ease into it. It's very important that you do.

Basketball

Like the three sports we just considered, basketball has interruptions built into it. Penalties and free throws can stop the action for several minutes at a time. The most "cardiovascular" basketball game would be one played without a single free throw, one with people running up and down the court every minute of the game. It's a very demanding game — while something is going on.

Besides the "start-stop" problem that basketball shares with other sports, the game can range from a full-scale, full-court game with ten players, officials, and fans to casual dribbling and basket shooting. At either extreme, you have limitations placed on basketball as a good cardiovascular exercise. Ironically, the more organized the game, the more starts, stops, time-outs, and rest periods there are.

If you decide to use basketball as an alternative, the best thing to do is to set up a game that is not timed, with no free-throws, jump-balls, or other pauses in the action. The exercise will then be sustained.

Uninterrupted basketball, however, requires the kind of stamina you need for handball. Just because you played it well 20 years ago does not mean you can take it up again without some pre-conditioning. Be sure you are in reasonably good shape before you get yourself into a strenuous game.

When you reach that point, you should aim for a workout on the basketball court that will last between 20 minutes and one hour and which will keep you moving constantly. If you can get enough people together for a game, fine. If you can't — and one of the disadvantages is not being able to round up enough players — then play by yourself. Dribble up and down the court, shoot baskets, keep moving. You may be a little lonely out there on that big court all by yourself, but you're keeping yourself healthy.

Rating
The
Running
Shoes

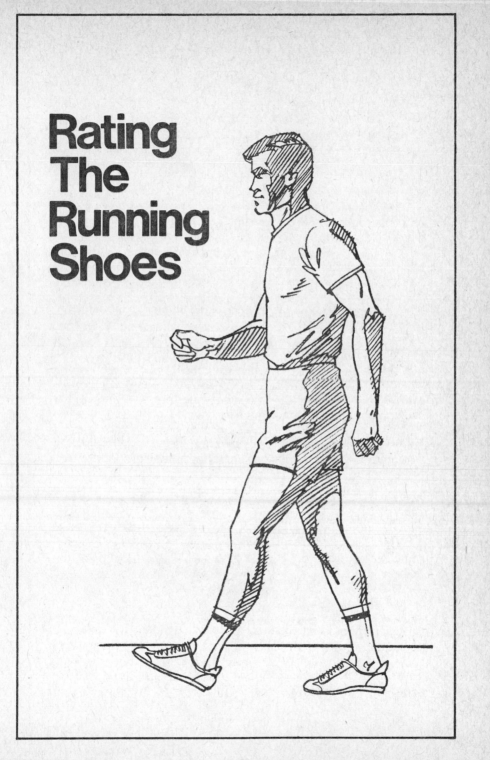

Running Shoes

SHOES ARE without doubt the most important equipment a runner owns. You can cover just as much territory in old shorts and a sweatshirt as you can in an expensive designer outfit, but a good pair of shoes means the difference between success and failure.

The feet of a runner take a lot of punishment and protecting them helps you to avoid injuries. In an ideal world, perhaps, we could all run barefoot through meadows, using our feet as they were meant to be used. Reality is different. Most of us have worn shoes from early childhood and our feet are accustomed to them. In addition, we do our running for the most part on pavement, hard roads, or packed-down tracks — all much rougher on the feet than springy grass.

There are, as always, exceptions to this rule. Abebe Bikila, the famous Ethiopian marathoner, won his Olympic Gold Medal by running barefoot through the streets of Rome. This astounding performance should be admired but not copied. All the authorities agree that shoes are the one item you should not skimp on. "Nothing, in fact," says Bob Anderson, founder and publisher of *Runner's World,* "is as important as a good pair of running shoes." He considers shoes so vital to successful running that his magazine devotes an entire issue each year to a comprehensive evaluation of the various brands on the market. Buy the best pair of shoes you can afford. They are an excellent investment.

Where To Buy Shoes

Only a few years ago, it was difficult to find shoes designed specifically for running. Most people had to be content with tennis shoes, sneakers, or other "sport" shoes. Today the situation is different. There are many excellent models designed for running that are readily available. Ordinary sports stores, some department and shoe stores, and shops catering specifically to runners carry the kinds of shoes you want.

The problem with these stores is that you may not be able to find one that carries the one brand you really want. If you live outside a metropolitan area or in an area where running is not yet popular, you are likely to become frustrated. The names and addresses of the major manufacturers are listed at the end of this chapter. Write or call them to find out what stores in your vicinity carry their products.

Another possibility is a mail-order dealer. Although you will not be able to inspect or try on the shoes before purchasing, in almost all cases you can return the shoes if you are not happy with them. Charles Kuntzleman, for example, buys all his shoes by mail and has encountered no problems. "Be sure to send them pencil tracings of your feet along with the size," he cautions. "When you get the shoes, try them on as soon as they arrive, walk around the house in them, and run in place. If the fit is not right or there is some other feature that makes them impractical for your feet or your running, send them back immediately." Don't wear the shoes outside, however, or you will not be able to return them.

Selecting Your Shoes

Finding exactly the right shoes can be a bit complicated. There are so many brands on the market that it is difficult to know which to choose. Personal preference plays a large part. As Jack Batten remarks, "Whatever fits and works for Jogger A may torment Jogger B." Nonetheless, there are certain guidelines that will help you make the right choice.

Fit

The first thing to remember is that *your* feet, not the experts', are going to wear the shoes. No matter how marvelous the

Running Shoes

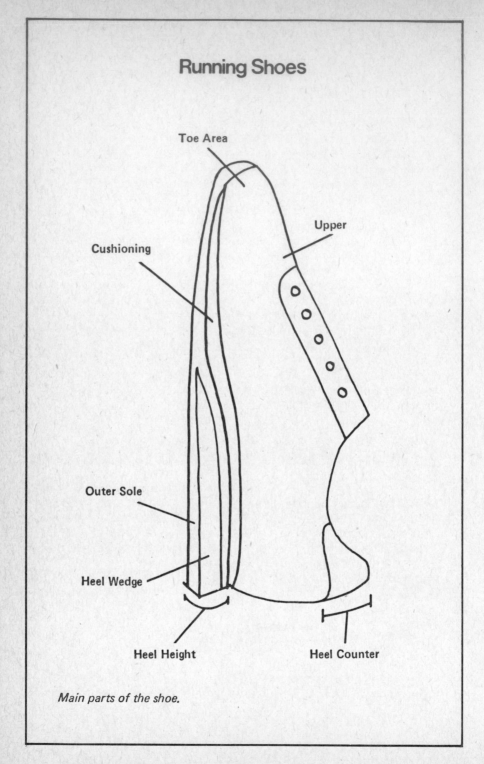

Main parts of the shoe.

Running Shoes

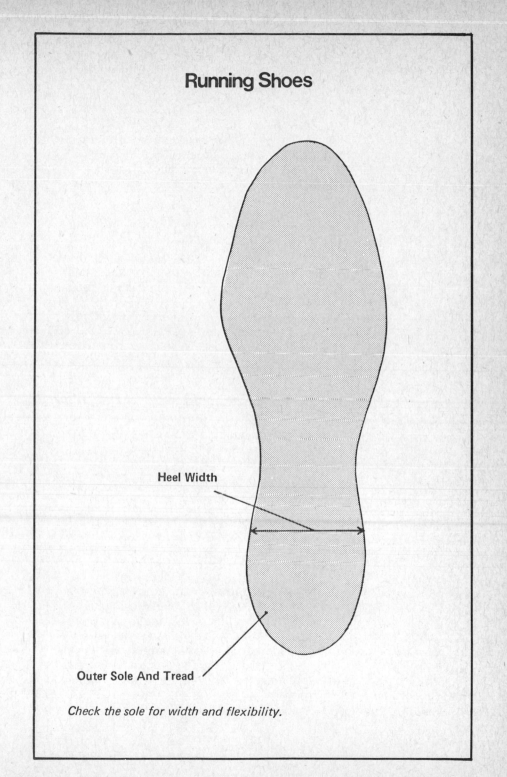

Heel Width

Outer Sole And Tread

Check the sole for width and flexibility.

design, if it isn't right for you, it's a waste of money. Your feet, like your fingerprints, are individual and you should make your selection with that in mind. The American Indians expressed a great truth when they said that, to understand another person, you must "walk a mile in his moccasins."

Begin by making an outline drawing of your feet. Simply place each foot on a piece of paper and trace around it. Since your left foot may be larger or smaller than your right foot, it's a good idea to trace both. When you go to the store, compare the bottom of each shoe to your tracings. How closely do the shoes conform to your feet? Are they wide enough across the ball and toe? Are they long enough?

Wear your running socks when trying the shoes on. If you plan to wear two pairs, as many runners do, wear both.

Check the toe area with special care. When you run, your foot will slide forward inside the shoe. Allow about three-fourths of an inch between your toe and the front of the shoe. Too snug a fit can cause undue pressure and blisters. Make sure your toes have enough room to spread out a little. Cramped toes cause problems.

Walk around the store and run in place for a minute to test for comfort. Even if the shoes are your size, they may not fit as well as they should.

Support

Because the runner hits the ground so many times during the course of a single run, the cumulative effect of these impacts is great. Most Americans have less than perfect feet that require good support in order to stand the rigors of running. Most shoes designed for running offer some measure of support, but it may not be sufficient for you. If the arch support in an otherwise excellent shoe seems inadequate, you can add foam rubber supports yourself. These devices are readily available. Good built-in support is preferable, however.

Weight

Ordinary running shoes vary considerably (up to 25%) in weight. The extra weight of the heavier shoes can become burdensome on a long run, so we recommend purchasing the lightest shoes you can find that have all the other features you need. Weight, by the way, is one of the differences between training flats (regular running shoes) and racing flats (shoes designed for speed and competitive running). Unless you are an experienced runner, stay with the heavier training flats.

Flexibility

Flexibility is one of the most important factors in judging a shoe. Unless the sole bends easily, your feet will suffer. Many injuries are caused by shoes that are too stiff. Bend the shoes back and forth to test pliability.

The Sole

Soles are all made of rubber but they vary a great deal in design. The sole must provide protection and cushioning while remaining flexible — no easy thing to accomplish. Most manufacturers solve the problem by providing double soles: a tough outer layer to resist impact and one, two, or more softer layers inside to cushion the feet and absorb shocks. This combination is definitely better than either hard or soft soles alone.

Treads are another distinctive feature. The trend today is toward the "waffle" tread which has a series of raised grippers designed to provide better traction. Originally intended for running on soft dirt and grass, the waffle is now being used for hard surfaces as well. A number of patterns, including square, round, star-shaped, and triangular grippers, are offered by different companies. Because the shock of impact is borne by the grippers rather than the whole foot, a waffle tread probably provides more cushioning than a flat tread. Pending further evidence, tread is largely a matter of personal preference.

Spikes are used primarily by racers. Although spikes may be helpful if you plan to do a great deal of bad-weather running over ice, they do increase the impact of each step and can be jarring. We do not recommend them for anyone but serious competitive runners.

The Heel

A poorly constructed heel can be the start of many problems. Narrow heels were popular in the past, but today most runners look for fairly wide heels that provide better stability. The heel of the shoe should hold the heel of your foot snugly without discomfort.

The height and depth of the heel are also important. Most authorities agree that a moderately elevated heel is best. Since Americans are accustomed to heels on their everyday shoes, the muscles at the back of our legs have shortened. Running tightens these muscles even more and an elevated heel reduces the amount of stretching required of them. Make sure the top of the heel hits the back of your foot at a comfortable level. If it is too low there will not be enough support and if it is too high you may develop blisters. Compare the depth of the heel with those on your regular shoes. The heel counter, the piece at the back of the shoe which supports the heel and Achilles tendon, should be firm and comfortable.

The Uppers

The uppers are the part of the shoe that give it its distinctive appearance. Resist the temptation to judge a shoe by its color or sportiness. Function is more important. The upper must be firm enough to stabilize the foot and soft enough on the inside so that it isn't irritating. Avoid shoes with thick seams that may rub against the foot, causing chafing.

Good running shoes offer you a choice of nylon, leather, or combination uppers. Serious runners like nylon uppers because they are lightweight, permit air circulation, and are water-resistant. They are also easier to clean — most nylon shoes can be tossed into a washing machine.

How Many Shoes Do You Need?

If you can afford it, owning two pairs of shoes is probably a good idea. Wear them on alternate runs. You may prefer to have one pair for ordinary running and one pair designed for bad-weather running. The extra pair is really a luxury rather than a necessity, however.

It is important to purchase new shoes before your old ones are completely worn out. Wear the new shoes on shorter runs to break them in. By the time your old ones are ready to be discarded, the new ones will be comfortable.

Rating The Shoes

We have evaluated the shoes now on the market and selected those that scored best in terms of the factors we have discussed. All the shoes here are excellent choices and you can select any of them with confidence. The listings within categories are alphabetical. The Highly Recommended shoes, for example, are comparable and you can pick the one that suits your own tastes and needs best. In many cases only minor differences separate the Also Recommended shoes from the Highly Recommended shoes.

Training Flats

Most runners will purchase training flats or basic running shoes. Until recently, women had little choice and were forced to cope with ill-fitting men's shoes. The new popularity of running, however, has encouraged manufacturers to produce first-rate shoes designed for the smaller, narrower feet of women. It is no longer necessary to settle for second-best.

HIGHLY RECOMMENDED TRAINING FLATS FOR MEN

Adidas Runner

Although expensive, Adidas shoes are worth the money because of their high-quality workmanship. The Runner is the top-of-the-line model that features a three-layered sole (at forefoot and heel) for extra cushioning. The tread is a waffle pattern designed for better traction. The new wider heel, introduced last year, is a definite plus. The wide heel has an outside groove to reduce impact shock. A nylon mesh upper provides good air circulation. The Runner is not the most flexible shoe, but it scores very high on strength and durability. Unfortunately, it is available in only one width so it will not be suitable for all runners.

Sizes: 5 to 15
Widths: One standard width
Suggested Retail Price: $40.95

Brooks Vantage

The Vantage won first place in *Runner's World's* annual evalua-

Running Shoes

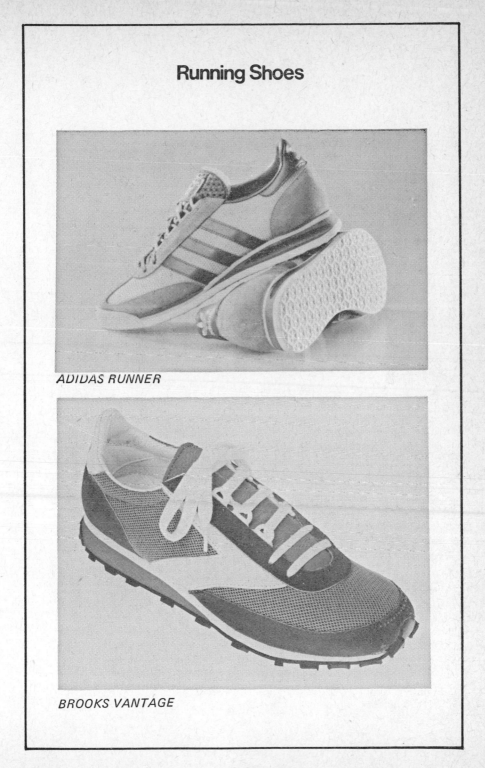

ADIDAS RUNNER

BROOKS VANTAGE

tion, a fact that should impress any runner. A number of features contribute to this high rating. A special "varus wedge," as Brooks calls it, tilts the feet slightly outward to compensate for the twisting action of the feet when running. Shock absorption is excellent because of the layered sole (two layers under the forefoot and three under the heel). The tread has "racing" studs but is still a training flat rather than a racing flat. Perhaps the best feature of the Vantage is the special innersole that molds itself to the runner's foot, providing excellent support. Nylon mesh uppers provide good air circulation. The only major disadvantage is that the sole is less durable than you would expect on a quality product.

Sizes: 4 to 13
Widths: Narrow, Medium, and Wide
Suggested Retail Price: $34.40

Etonic Street Fighter

The Street Fighter offers more than an encouraging name. Perhaps its best feature is the first-class built-in arch support. The one-piece heel/arch support is designed to compensate for the heel flattening caused by years of walking. The heel provides good shock absorption, but the forefoot is not cushioned as well. The waffle-tread sole scores very high on durability as does the nylon-and-suede upper.

Sizes: 6 to 13
Widths: Narrow, Medium, and Wide
Suggested Retail Price: $29.95

New Balance 320

Although the 320 does not score as high as some other models, it has one major advantage that moves it into the Highly Recommended category — it comes in all the standard widths of regular shoes. This makes it easy to obtain the proper fit. The 320 also offers good shock absorption, particularly at the extra-wide heel. The one-piece polyester-and-suede upper has a padded tongue for greater comfort and is quite flexible. The

Running Shoes

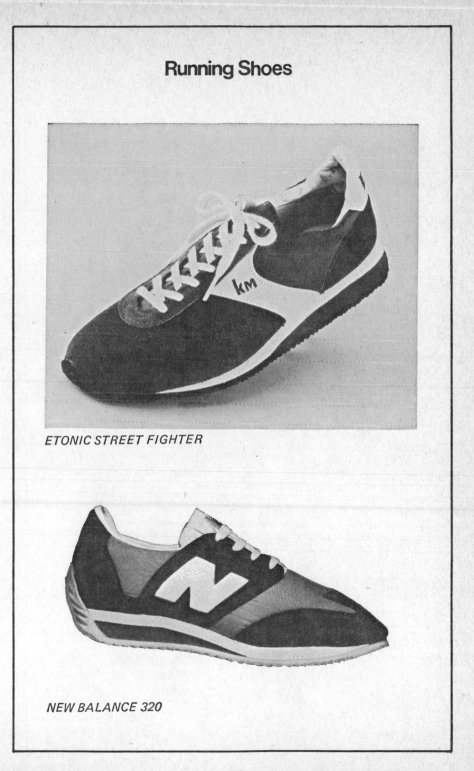

ETONIC STREET FIGHTER

NEW BALANCE 320

padded heel counter provides excellent support. Sole durability, however, is below average. It has a flat tread.

Sizes: 3½ to 15
Widths: AA to EEEE
Suggested Retail Price: $29.95

Nike Waffle Trainer

As you might expect from its name, the Waffle Trainer possesses the unique square tread pattern introduced by Nike in 1975 and since adapted by other manufacturers. The shoe is particularly good for running over rough terrain. The forefoot provides excellent shock absorption but the heel, despite four layers of cushioning, does not. The upper is nylon accented with suede. The Waffle Trainer, along with the New Balance 320, is about 10% lighter than the other Highly Recommended shoes, making it suitable for some racing. Despite this lighter weight, it offers good support and durability.

Sizes: 3 to 13
Widths: One standard width
Suggested Retail Price: $29.95

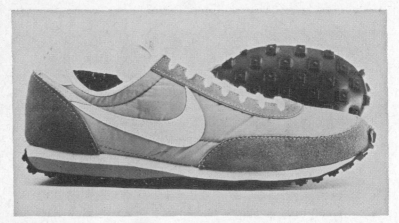

NIKE WAFFLE TRAINER

Running Shoes

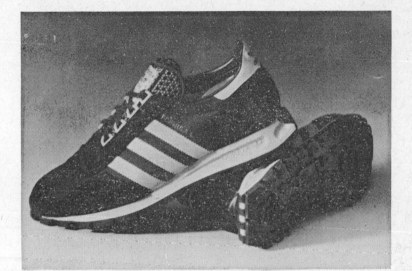

ADIDAS FORMULA 1

ALSO RECOMMENDED TRAINING FLATS FOR MEN

Adidas Formula 1

This odd-looking shoe has a heel that juts out in back. It is supposed to provide better shock absorption and stability, but the Formula 1 scores fairly low on these qualities. Forefoot shock absorption, however, is excellent. This is a relatively heavy shoe, but sole and upper durability are only average. The high heel lift is designed to relieve strain on the Achilles tendon, a definite plus. An expanded rubber arch provides good support. The upper is leather and the tread is a waffle pattern that Adidas calls a "racing profile."

Sizes: 5 to 15
Widths: One standard width
Suggested Retail Price: $39.95

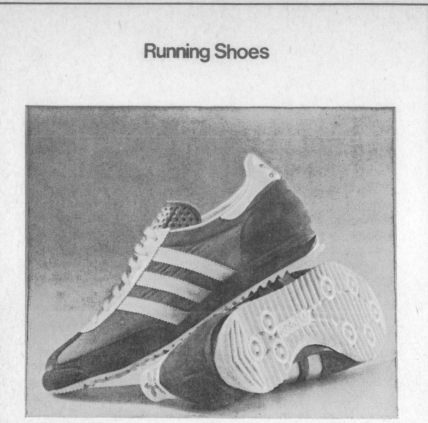

ADIDAS SL-72

Adidas SL-72 and SL-76

These two models are very similar. The main difference between them is color, although the SL-72 is slightly more flexible. Suction-cup treads provide good traction. The wide heel has a shock-absorbing groove and the three-layered heel wedge cushions effectively. Forefront cushioning is less adequate. The SL-76 has a higher heel lift than its companion model. The nylon upper is very lightweight and comfortable.

Sizes: 5 to 15
Widths: One standard width
Suggested Retail Price: $33.95

Running Shoes

Brooks Delta

The Delta resembles the higher-ranked Vantage but has a thinner sole and a less porous nylon upper. The sole rates an excellent for shock absorption but scores low on durability. The tread is spiked. A built-in arch provides good support. The innersole is contoured and comfortable.

Sizes: 4 to 13
Widths: Narrow, Medium, and Wide
Suggested Retail Price: $28.80

Brooks Villanova

Perhaps the most attractive feature of this medium-weight shoe is its low price. The Villanova also receives high marks for

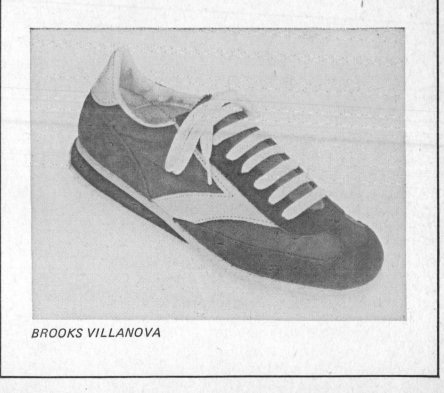

BROOKS VILLANOVA

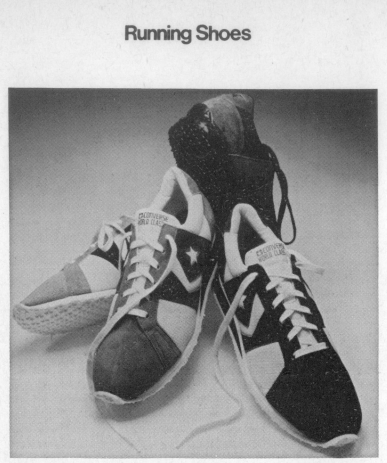

CONVERSE WORLD CLASS TRAINER

flexibility and shock absorption. The suction-cup tread provides good traction but is below average in durability. The upper is nylon.

Sizes: 4 to 13
Widths: Narrow, Medium, and Wide
Suggested Retail Price: $25.20

Converse World Class Trainer

This is a strong and durable shoe, but one less comfortable

than many of the other models. Despite a three-layered forefoot and a four-layered heel, the cushioning seems inadequate. On the other hand, the nylon mesh upper, trimmed with suede, is unusually strong. A star-pattern tread provides good traction.

Sizes: 4 to 13
Widths: Narrow, Medium, and Wide
Suggested Retail Price: $28.00

Etonic KM

Like the Street Fighter, the KM offers excellent heel shock absorption and arch support but does less well on forefoot shock absorption. It also scores poorly on the durability of the nylon upper. Because of the good support it offers and its superior flexibility, however, the KM has a high overall rating. The sole is a star-pattern design.

Sizes: 6 to 13
Widths: Narrow, Medium, and Wide
Suggested Retail Price: $27.95

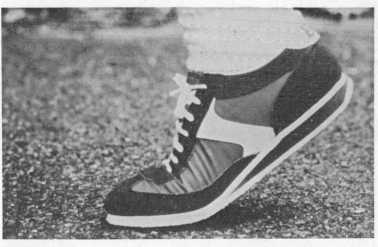

ETONIC KM

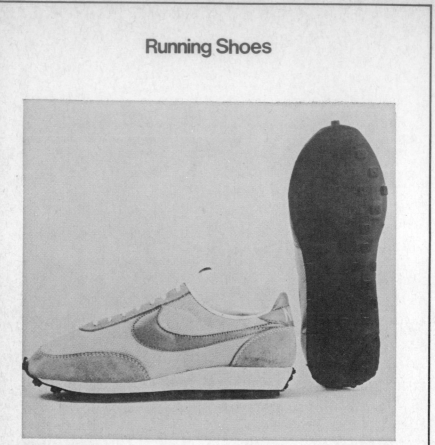

NIKE LD-1000V

Nike LD-1000V

This shoe is highly regarded but loses points because of its high cost and poor flexibility. The LD-1000V receives superior scores for shock absorption (forefoot and heel) and support. The sole is an extra-deep waffle tread that offers good cushioning and protection. The solid-rubber inserts at stress points in the heel are another asset. The polyester mesh upper is excellent.

Sizes: 3 to 13
Widths: One standard width
Suggested Retail Price: $39.95

Running Shoes

Pony California

This is a strong, comfortable shoe that earns high marks for shock absorption (forefoot and heel). There are three layers under the forefoot and four under the heel. The tread is a waffle pattern. The upper, made of nylon mesh, is comfortable but not as durable as those of many other models. It also scores fairly low on flexibility.

Sizes: 3 to 13
Widths: Medium only
Suggested Retail Price: $28.00

Pony Racer

This heavyweight shoe offers a waffle tread designed for shock absorption and a special innersole that adapts to the shape of

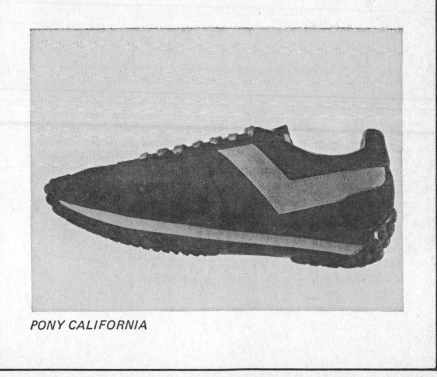

PONY CALIFORNIA

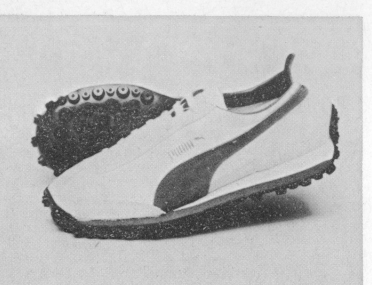

PUMA EASY RIDER

the foot. Traction is excellent. The upper is nylon mesh trimmed with suede.

Sizes: 6½ to 12
Widths: Narrow, Medium, and Wide
Suggested retail price: $34.00

Puma Easy Rider

The Easy Rider rates an excellent for support and forefoot cushioning, but it is below average in heel shock absorption. The studded tread is a very deep waffle for traction. The nylon upper is strong and comfortable. This is a real heavyweight.

Sizes: 3 to 14
Widths: One standard size
Suggested Retail Price: $40.00

Running Shoes

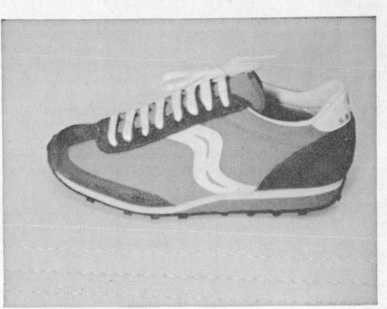

SAUCONY GRIPPER

Saucony Gripper

This waffle tread offers excellent traction and the flared heel provides stability. Although forefoot cushioning could be improved, heel cushioning is among the best on the market. The nylon mesh upper is durable and comfortable.

Sizes: 6 to 13
Widths: Medium only
Suggested Retail Price: $24.95

Saucony Hornet

The Hornet's low price, light weight, and excellent heel construction make it a bargain. Sole durability, however, is only average. The tread is a herringbone pattern. Both forefoot and

Running Shoes

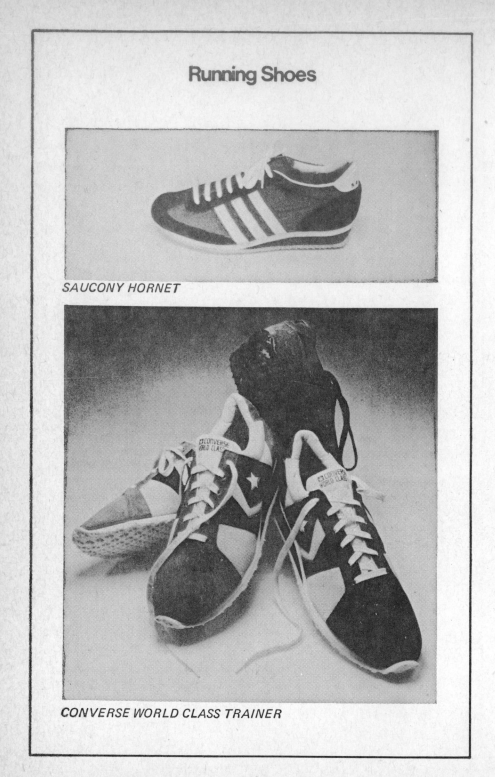

SAUCONY HORNET

CONVERSE WORLD CLASS TRAINER

heel score well in shock absorption. The upper is nylon with vinyl trim.

Sizes: 3 to 14
Width: Narrow, Medium, and Wide
Suggested Retail Price: $22.95

HIGHLY RECOMMENDED TRAINING FLATS FOR WOMEN

Brooks Victress

This top-of-the-line model is lightweight but durable. The suction-cup tread provides traction and stability and is enhanced by the wide, cushioned heel. The two-layer forefoot and three-layer heel give the Victress excellent shock absorption, an important factor in judging a shoe. Heel cushioning is particularly good. The Victress also offers good arch support. Although the nylon-and-suede upper gives only average breathability, it is rugged and designed for wear and tear.

Sizes: 4 to 10
Widths: One standard width
Suggested Retail Price: $28.80

Converse World Class Trainer

This shoe was developed for the serious woman runner. It is extremely lightweight but handles the stresses of hard running quite well. The tread design, a star waffle pattern, provides effective traction and the wide heel gives stability. The upper is nylon mesh trimmed with suede and is exceptionally durable as well as comfortable, a fact bound to please a dedicated runner. The flared heel wedge and full-length sponge padding provide good shock absorption. A contoured arch cushion supports the foot well.

Sizes: 5 to 10
Widths: Narrow, Medium, and Wide
Suggested Retail Price: $28.00

Running Shoes

Etonic Street Fighter

The women's Street Fighter is more than a scaled-down version of the men's shoe. The excellent one-piece heel/arch support is comparable to that of the men's model. The star tread pattern provides good traction and the sole is extremely rugged. The heel is not particularly wide but is higher than that of most other shoes. The nylon-and-suede upper is designed for hard use and holds up well.

Sizes: 5 to 10
Widths: Narrow and Medium
Suggested Retail Price: $29.95

Nike Lady Waffle Trainer

The Lady Waffle Trainer offers many of the fine features found on the men's models, but is built on a narrow last which Nike

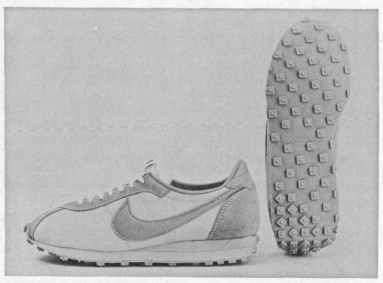

NIKE LADY WAFFLE TRAINER

Running Shoes

feels is better suited to the bone structure of most women. The deep waffle tread and layered sole (two layers under the forefoot and three under the heel) provide excellent shock absorption. The heel is tapered for comfort and arch support is good. The upper is made of nylon and suede and is tops for strength and durability. Breathability, however, is inferior to that of other top-quality shoes.

Sizes: 4 to 10
Widths: One standard width
Suggested Retail Price: $29.95

Tiger Tigress

This medium-weight shoe combines comfort with durability. The herringbone tread provides less traction than many of the waffle patterns but is extremely durable. It holds up well over rough terrain. The relatively narrow heel is a drawback because

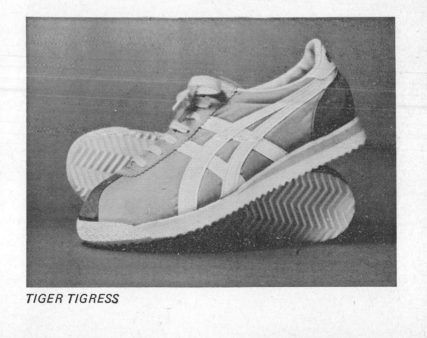

TIGER TIGRESS

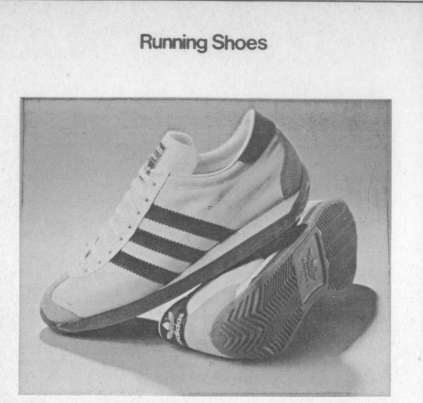

ADIDAS COUNTRY GIRL

it is less stable than the wider heel on other models. The upper, however, is especially good. The nylon material promotes air circulation and the padding adapts nicely to the contours of the foot.

Sizes: 3 to 10
Widths: One standard width
Suggested Retail Price: $28.95

ALSO RECOMMENDED TRAINING FLATS FOR WOMEN

Adidas Country Girl

Unlike most shoes, the Country Girl is leather. This makes it unusually durable and strong but adds considerably to its

Running Shoes

weight. The tread is a herringbone pattern. The uppers resist wet and cold, an advantage to the bad-weather runner.

Sizes: 5 to 14
Widths: One standard width
Suggested Retail Price: $29.95

Brooks Women's Villanova

This is very similar to the men's model, differing primarily in sizing and color. Like its companion model, it offers many fine features at a low price. Its most notable assets are good shock absorption and a suction-cup tread. The upper is nylon and suede.

Sizes: 4 to 10
Widths: One standard width
Suggested Retail Price: $25.20

Etonic KM

The KM, like the excellent Street Fighter, offers a heel/arch

BROOKS WOMEN'S VILLANOVA

Running Shoes

support that is superior. The star pattern tread provides good traction and heel cushioning is first-rate.

Sizes: 5 to 10
Widths: Narrow and Medium
Suggested Retail Price: $27.95

New Balance 320

Once again, the 320 merits high praise for the range of widths available. Almost every woman will be able to obtain an excellent fit. In addition, the 320 offers good shock absorption and superior heel cushioning. The tread is a herringbone and the high heel lift is a plus. This medium-weight shoe has a nylon upper.

Sizes: 3½ to 10½
Widths: AAAA to EEEE
Suggested Retail Price: $27.95

Puma Rockette

Despite its overly cute name, the Rockette is a heavy-duty running shoe with a contoured tread for traction. The sole combines flexibility with good shock absorption. The upper is nylon and suede.

Sizes: 4 to 10
Widths: One standard width
Suggested Retail Price: $26.00

Saucony Ms. Gripper

This medium-weight shoe has a waffle tread for traction and scores well on shock absorption. The upper is nylon mesh and suede.

Sizes: 4 to 10
Widths: One standard width
Suggested Retail Price: $24.95

Running Shoes

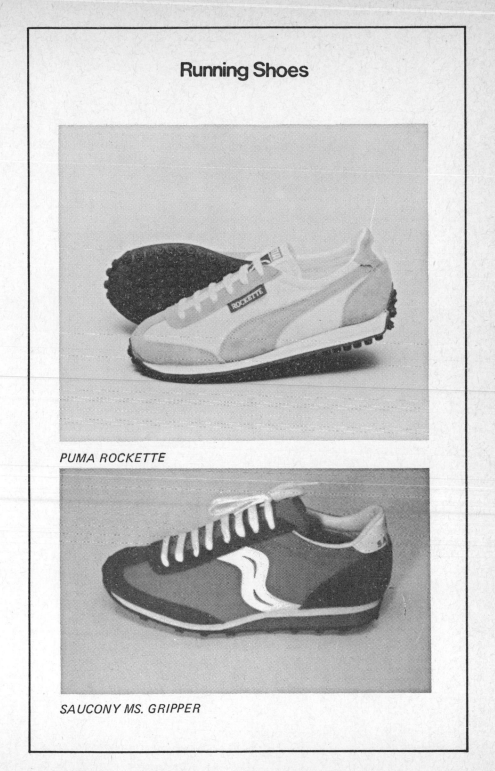

PUMA ROCKETTE

SAUCONY MS. GRIPPER

Racing Flats

Racing flats are designed for speed. They are lighter in weight than training flats and usually have thinner soles. You need not be a track star before you buy a pair, but you should be a serious runner who races against time (your own or that of others). The beginner is better off with training flats. Spiked shoes are definitely for competitive runners and are not included in these ratings.

Men have a wide variety of racing flats to choose from, but the selection is much more limited for women. This is particularly unfortunate because it is estimated that more than 30% of the serious runners in the United States are female. Only a few years ago, however, there were only a few training flats designed for women. In the near future, manufacturers of racing flats may catch up with the demand as well.

HIGHLY RECOMMENDED RACING FLATS FOR MEN

Adidas Arrow

The Arrow proves that it is possible to produce a low-cost shoe without sacrificing quality. It is lightweight but very strong and durable. The deep waffle sole provides excellent traction and good shock absorption and flexibility. The upper, made of nylon trimmed with leather, scores lower on strength and breathability. The heel is relatively narrow, but the lift is higher than average.

Sizes: 3 to 13
Widths: One standard width
Suggested Retail Price: $23.95

Brooks Texan

The Texan is a medium-weight shoe that scores well in every area except flexibility where it rates only average. Like the Van-

Running Shoes

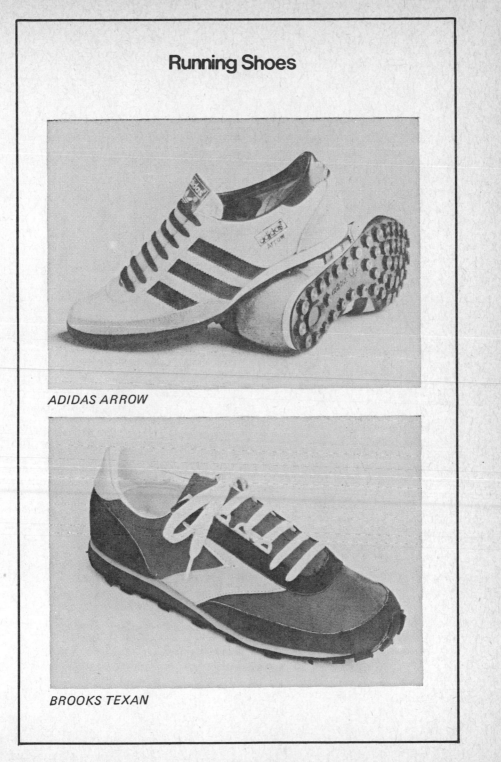

ADIDAS ARROW

BROOKS TEXAN

tage training flat, the Texan has the special Brooks innersole that molds itself to the contours of the foot, offering excellent support. The flared heel adds stability and the waffle tread provides good traction. The three-layered cushioning at the heel makes the Texan rate high in shock absorption. The upper is nylon trimmed with suede and is designed for hard running.

Sizes: 4 to 13
Widths: Narrow, Medium, and Wide
Suggested Retail Price: $28.80

Converse World Class Marathoner

Long-known for athletic shoes, Converse entered the racing flat market with the World Class Marathoner. It is very lightweight

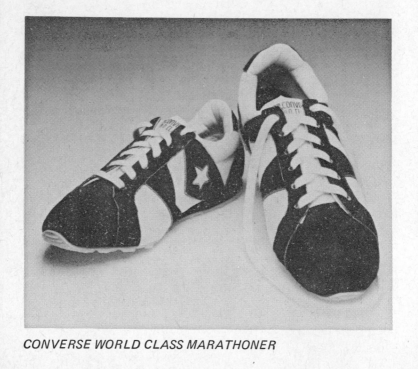

CONVERSE WORLD CLASS MARATHONER

Running Shoes

and receives top scores for flexibility. The star-pattern tread does not provide as much traction as some other models, but is quite durable. Shock absorption is better than average and the nylon mesh upper offers exceptional breathability.

Sizes: 4 to 14
Widths: Narrow, Medium, and Wide
Suggested Retail Price: $32.00

Nike Elite

Charles Kuntzleman says that the Elite is the finest racing flat on the market. The panel of experts at *Runner's World* agrees.

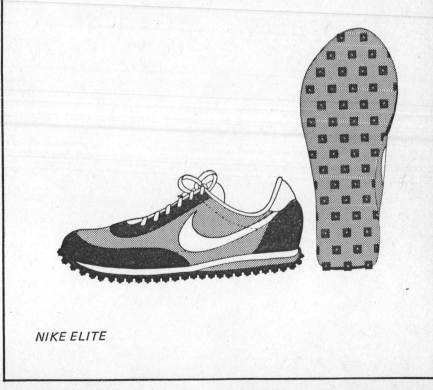

NIKE ELITE

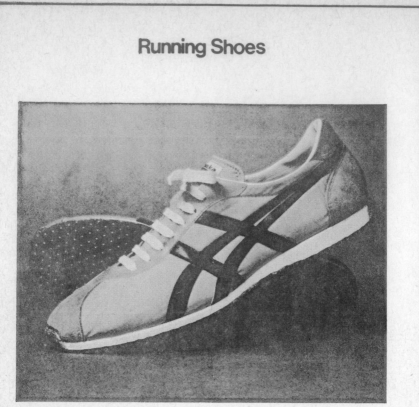

TIGER JAYHAWK

Exceptionally fine shock absorption (two layers under the forefoot and three under the heel) accounts for much of the enthusiasm. In addition, the waffle tread offers excellent traction and durability. The upper, made of nylon and suede, is very strong and breathability is first-rate. The only disadvantages are the relatively high price, lack of width selection, and below-average flexibility.

Sizes: 3 to 13
Widths: One standard width
Suggested Retail Price: $33.95

Tiger Jayhawk

The Jayhawk has been around a lot longer than most of its competition. It scores high in flexibility and shock absorption.

Running Shoes

The crepe sole offers adequate traction and both forefront and heel are cushioned by three layers of rubber. The heel is relatively narrow, but the nylon upper is rugged.

Sizes: 4 to 13
Widths: One standard width
Suggested Retail Price: $28.95

ALSO RECOMMENDED RACING FLATS FOR MEN

Brooks Floridian

A built-in arch support and good heel cushioning are the strong points of this model. The high heel lift is also a fine feature. The suction-cup tread provides good traction. The nylon upper, however, is only average in strength.

Sizes: 4 to 13
Widths: One standard width
Suggested Retail Price: $25.20

E. B. Boston

This is extremely lightweight, yet the sole scores high on durability. The waffle tread offers good traction and heel cushioning is excellent. Forefoot cushioning, however, is inferior to those of most of the other models. The contoured suspension arch is very comfortable. The upper is nylon and not as strong as it might be.

Sizes: 3½ to 13
Widths: One standard width
Suggested Retail Price: $29.99

E. B. Marathon

This leather shoe is more expensive than most. Sole durability is excellent and so is flexibility. The waffle tread provides good

Running Shoes

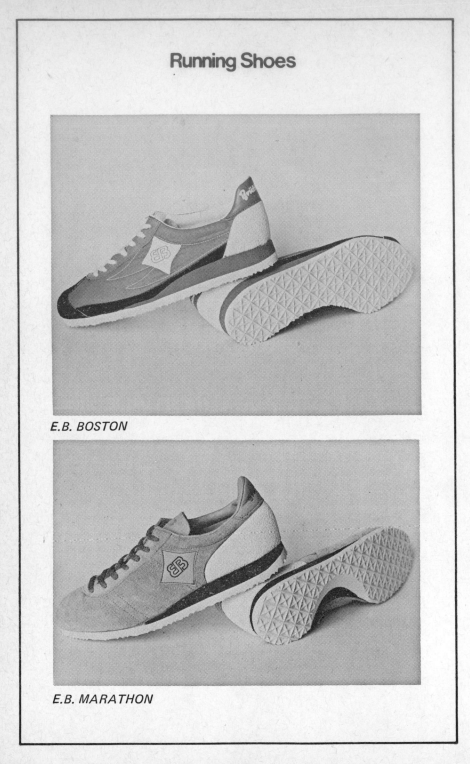

E.B. BOSTON

E.B. MARATHON

Running Shoes

traction. The Marathon has the contoured suspension arch found on the Boston. Forefoot shock absorption is poor.

Sizes: 3½ to 14
Widths: One standard width
Suggested Retail Price: $37.99

New Balance Super Comp

A bit on the heavy side for a racing flat, the Super Comp is both comfortable and durable. Shock absorption is excellent. The flat tread offers surprisingly good traction. The polyester mesh upper is one of the shoe's best features. The great variety of widths available make the proper fit easy to obtain.

Sizes: 3½ to 15
Widths: AA to EEEE
Suggested Retail Price: $29.95

Nike Sting

The Sting is a durable shoe that offers excellent shock absorp-

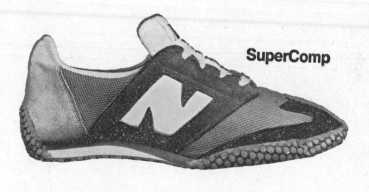

SuperComp

NEW BALANCE SUPER COMP

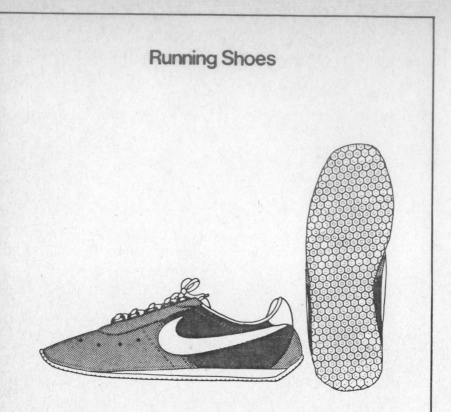

NIKE STING

tion. The flat tread provides good traction and the wide heel is a definite asset. The nylon-and-suede upper is rugged.

Sizes: 3 to 13
Widths: One standard width
Suggested Retail Price: $36.95

Nike Waffle Racer

One of the lightest racing flats around, the Waffle Racer scores low on sole durability. It does provide excellent shock absorption and is quite flexible. The waffle tread offers good traction. The upper is nylon trimmed with suede.

Sizes: 3 to 13
Widths: One standard width
Suggested Retail Price: $29.95

Running Shoes

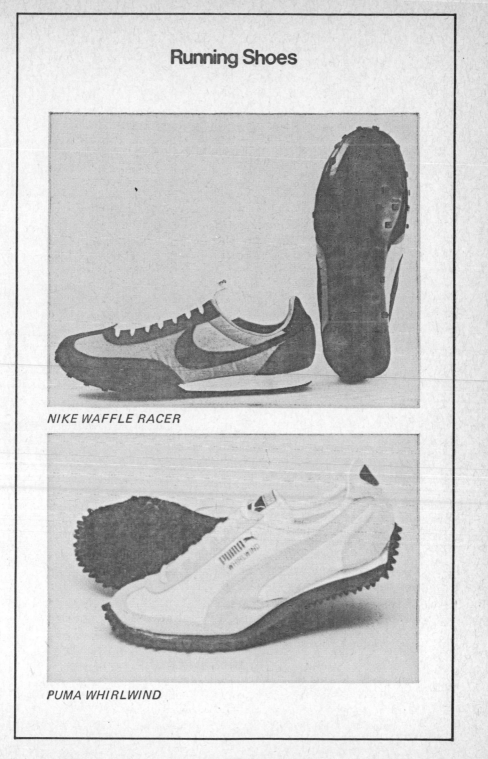

NIKE WAFFLE RACER

PUMA WHIRLWIND

TIGER OHBORI

Puma Whirlwind

The Whirlwind offers great shock absorption, an important point in its favor. The waffle tread sole, however, scores low on flexibility and durability. The nylon upper, trimmed with suede, is more rugged. Although the Whirlwind is rather heavy for a racing flat, it is extremely comfortable.

Sizes: 3 to 13
Widths: One standard width
Suggested Retail Price: $28.00

Tiger Ohbori

Another old favorite in the running world, the Ohbori continues to merit its popularity. Although it scores low on sole durability,

Running Shoes

as do most lightweight shoes, it does well on shock absorption. Forefoot cushioning is particularly good. The nylon upper is very rugged and the flat suction-cup tread is effective. Its heel may be too narrow for some runners.

Sizes: 5 to 13
Widths: One standard width
Suggested Retail Price: $37.95

HIGHLY RECOMMENDED RACING FLATS FOR WOMEN

Converse World Class Marathoner

This is a fairly expensive shoe, but it does give you quite a bit for your money. Despite its very lightweight construction, the Marathoner is durable. The relatively high heel lift provides excellent support, although shock absorption could be improved.

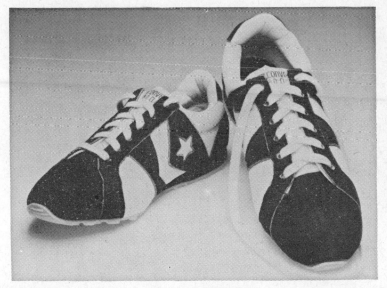

CONVERSE WORLD CLASS MARATHONER

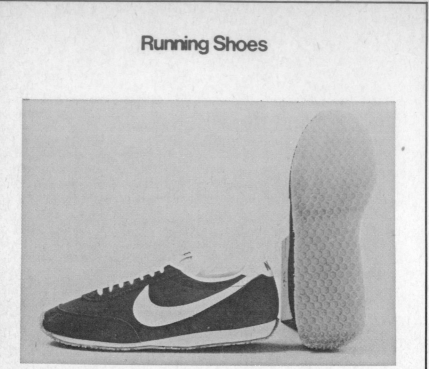

NIKE MIEKA

The star pattern tread offers good traction and the nylon mesh upper is rugged.

Sizes: 5 to 10
Widths: Narrow, Medium, and Wide
Suggested Retail Price: $32.00

Nike Mieka

The Mieka scores high because of the excellence of its heel construction and durability. The flat tread provides only average traction, but the layered sole is flexible. Shock absorption is outstanding. The nylon-and-suede upper offers only adequate breathability but is superior in strength and ruggedness. The foam rubber arch support is excellent and the wide heel adds stability.

Sizes: 4 to 10
Widths: One standard width
Suggested Retail Price: $27.95

Some Special Problems

As we stated earlier, feet are not alike. Neither are running habits. Some of the most common problems faced by runners with less-than-perfect feet are discussed below. If you are among these runners, you should look for some special features when you select your shoes. In many cases, shoes now on the market can solve, or at least minimize, your difficulties.

Feet That Roll Inward

Most human feet tend to roll inward when running. Extended running on feet that roll to an excessive degree can aggravate the condition and cause foot and leg problems. Look for shoes that offer balance and stability. Any shoe with a wide heel will help. The new "varus wedge" on shoes made by Brooks should be particularly useful. This special wedge is designed to compensate for inward rolling.

Morton's Toe

Morton's toe is not a disease but a matter of bone structure. The big toe is the longest on most feet and takes most of the stress. On some feet, however, the second toe, which is weaker, is the longest. Although many people never experience difficulties, others endure blisters and heel and leg strain as a result. Look for shoes with roomy toe areas that permit the foot to slide forward without undue pressure on the ends of the toes. The Formula 1 and the Country Girl, both by Adidas, rate high.

Unstable Heel

Sometimes called "loose ankles," this balancing problem can be overcome by wider heels. Most of the manufacturers are aware of this and narrow heels are losing popularity. The Adidas Runner and the New Balance 320 have the widest heels

Running Shoes

on men's flats and the Converse World Class Trainer and the Brooks Victress the widest on women's shoes.

Odd Widths

Hard-to-fit feet can be a real problem because so many running shoes come in one standard width. Even those that offer three widths may not fit properly. New Balance offers the greatest selection of widths of any major manufacturer (AA to EEEE for men and AAAA to EEEE for women).

MANUFACTURERS OF RECOMMENDED SHOES

Adidas USA Inc.
2382 Townsgate Road
Westlake Village, CA 91361
(805) 497-9575

Brooks Shoe Mfg. Co.
Factory and Terrace Streets
Hanover, PA 17331
(717) 632-1755

Converse Rubber Co.
55 Fordham Rd.
Wilmington, MA 01887
(617) 657-5735

E.B. Sport International
Lydiard Enterprise
Box 180
Basking Ridge, NJ 07920
(201) 234-9011

Etonic
Eaton Co.
147 Centre St.
Brockton, Mass. 02403
(617) 583-9100

Running Shoes

New Balance Athletic Shoes
38-42 Everett St.
Boston, Mass. 02134
(617) 783-4000

Nike
8285 S.W. Nimbus Ave.
Beaverton, OR 97005
(503) 641-6453

Pony Sports & Leisure Inc.
251 Park Ave. South
New York, NY 10010
(213) 533-9800

Puma
Beconta Inc.
50 Executive Blvd.
Elmsford, NY 10523
(914) 592-4444

Saucony Shoe Mfg. Co.
14 Peach St.
Kutztown, PA 19530
(215) 683-8711

Tiger
2052 Alton Ave.
Irvine, CA 92714
(714) 754-0451

Other Equipment

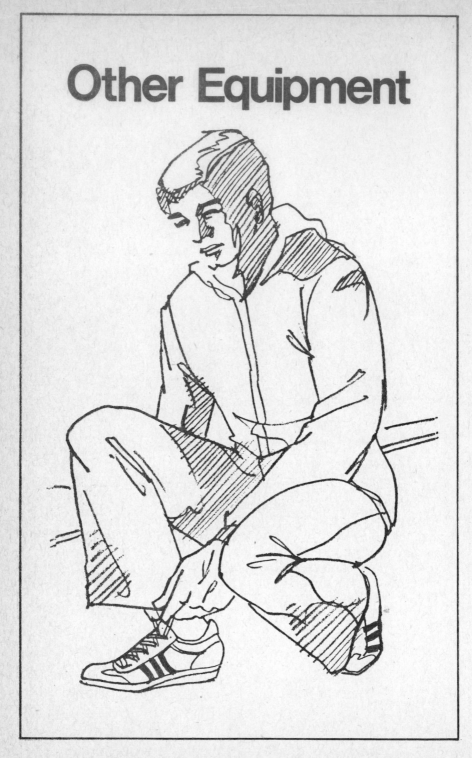

Other Equipment

IF YOU WENT to Detroit to watch new cars roll off the assembly line, perhaps one in 50 would look rather unfinished to you. It would have no chrome accents, no blue tint in the windshield, no radio, no power equipment, no accessories of any kind. Such a car is called a "stripped model."

The athletes who competed in the Olympics and other games of the ancient world were stripped models, too. Since the Greeks considered a splendid male body the most beautiful of earthly things, the competitors were all nude. In fact, our word gymnasium, a place for athletic activities, is derived from *gymnos,* the Greek word for naked.

Your neighbors, however, are apt to be a bit less enthusiastic about such goings on, so we suggest that you do your running in something besides shoes!

Clothes

Your outfit can be as stylish or as shabby as you like. Your main goal is not to coordinate the colors of your European tailored all-weather suit with your suede and nylon shoes, but your left foot with your right. We are not against fancy running outfits. No doubt they raise the spirits of the people who wear them, the people who watch them brightening up the landscape, and surely the people who sell them. Those dreary gray sweatsuits that have become a tradition for athletes may help the feet skip faster, but certainly not the heart. Maybe if the heart skips faster in those fancy, colorful clothes, the feet will follow.

We don't know. Whether you want to look like those stunning people from the pages of *Vogue* and the *Gentleman's Quarterly* or Marie Dressler and Wallace Beery is all the same to us, but you should pick the clothes you run in with two things in mind: comfort and the weather.

Running Suits

We've already talked about some of the medical hazards of running in the heat. The right kinds of clothes can reduce them.

Other Equipment

Wear something that will let the body "breathe" as much as possible. Wear as little as you can. Nylon or cotton running shorts are the best, with nylon probably the more comfortable of the two. Cotton can cause chafing, partly because it absorbs more perspiration than nylon and partly because the thicker cotton seams tend to irritate the thighs.

Cotton is the best material for the upper body in hot weather. It absorbs perspiration and is "cool," permitting perspiration to evaporate easily as you run.

Many male runners go shirtless, but if you prefer to run fully covered, running suits, sometimes called sweatsuits, are available in different materials and designs. There is no shortage of expensive fashions. But if you go this route, do not wear a running suit which is rubberized, plastic, or otherwise nonporous. In warm or hot weather you don't want heat and moisture to be trapped. You want it to circulate, escape, and keep your body cool. Those who imagine they are undergoing a kind of "Turkish bath" on the hoof are merely deluding themselves. They may perspire a lot more than someone running in shorts and lose water and weight momentarily, but they will promptly put both back on when they rush to the water fountain.

You want, instead, a suit that is porous, made either of cotton or of a combination of cotton and porous synthetic fiber. It should be loose-fitting, but not so loose as to impede your running.

In cold weather you don't want air to circulate or moisture to escape. You want to keep it from doing so. You reverse your hot weather strategy, constructing a personal heating system with your body as the furnace. To do that you must trap and hold the heated air your body continually generates by dressing in layers of clothing. The arrangement is very much like the insulation in your home: it holds in the heat generated by your heating system and keeps out the cold. The insulation forms a barrier that prevents heat and cold from passing in either direction through the ceiling and the walls. The layers of clothing trap air between them and hold it next to the body. The more you work, the warmer the air becomes. At the same time, these layers of warm air act as a barrier to the cold, with the help of a windbreaker, the best of which is usually made of nylon.

Whether you are dressing for summer or winter — a simple

Other Equipment

running suit for warm weather or assorted layers of clothing for cold weather — always make sure that you are a little "cold" in the clothes you are in when you step out of the door. You want to be sure that you won't find yourself uncomfortably warm in the middle of your run, loaded down with clothing you have to shed and carry by hand the rest of the way.

Socks

Some runners don't wear socks at all. They say that socks give them blisters. Others say just the opposite. They wear socks to keep from getting blisters. We recommend the use of socks, at least for most people. We've found that a pair of socks provides a little extra cushion between the skin of the feet and the soles of the running shoes that cuts down on blisters and other skin irritations. But we cannot ignore the simple truth that blisters and irritations of this kind depend entirely on the shoe and the foot that's in it. Heat causes friction and friction causes the blister. If the fit is so excellent without a sock that there is no friction and, therefore, no blister, we won't argue. You simply have to decide on the basis of your own experience and through the careful selection of the right shoe in the first place. It should be emphasized that it is better to buy a shoe that feels completely right on your foot than one that has been highly rated — by us or by anyone else.

In any case, running socks should be either cotton or wool. They absorb the most moisture and that, along with the comfort socks can give, is the main thing they are supposed to do. Some runners prefer cotton over wool, because wool, they say, itches. Again, it's an individual matter.

Less subjective, perhaps, is sock length. There are two basic lengths: anklets that reach to just above the shoe top and socks that go half-way up the calf. Anklets are better for summer running since they are cooler. But the calf-high variety is more suited to winter running because it offers greater protection.

Underwear

On long runs men can suffer irritation from jock straps, a problem which some runners have solved with an apparently satis-

Other Equipment

factory, if unusual, substitute — women's panties. Some manufacturers of running shorts have more or less followed that lead by designing "unisex" running shorts, worn by men and women alike, designed with a built-in support and made of nylon that will not rub, bind, or chafe.

Dr. Joan Ullyot, women's editor for *Runner's World,* recently raised an important question, especially when you consider all the advertising effort that goes into promoting all those fancy outfits with leg zippers, cute insignias, and color-coordinated stripes down the sleeve: "But what of underpinnings? Who is giving a thought to that non-visible, but essential part of the female runner's ensemble — the bra?"

She surveyed a group of marathoners who did agree on the characteristics they would like to see in the ideal bra: no metal fasteners, hooks, loops, or wires — nothing to rub and no seams at all. In short, a single-piece, all-stretch design made of a soft material such as cotton or nylon knit that could be pulled over the head and provide enough support to limit bouncing of the breasts.

Many runners, male as well as female, coat their nipples with Vaseline to reduce friction and irritation. This tip should be especially helpful to large-breasted women.

Caps, Masks, And Mittens

Caps—It has been estimated that a cap keeps in 80% of the body's heat during winter. Put a cap on the head and, in effect, you have capped the heat's escape route. You should wear a heavy knitted wool ski cap when you run in winter, especially one you can pull down over your ears.

If body heat is lost through the head, it is also gained through the head. The head is the first part of the body struck by the powerful rays of the summer sun. If you can control that onrush of heat attacking the head, you can help control your body temperature when you run in the summer. For this, it is a good practice to wear a lightweight cap, preferably one that is white or at least light-colored to deflect the sun's rays. This will help keep your head and, in turn, your body cool.

Masks — Your face is vulnerable to the bitter winds of winter

Other Equipment

and can become frostbitten if not adequately covered. Some runners have taken to wearing facemasks like those worn by skiers. If you wear one, it should be wool, and large enough to fit comfortably while permitting you to breathe easily. A ski mask can protect you from the cold and be conveniently rolled up to form a cap if you don't need it for your face.

But a mask is not an unmixed blessing to its owner. Perspiration and condensation of the breath can freeze into ice around the mouth and nostril area, not the most pleasant winter experience. Some runners have complained that the masks tend to congest the sinuses because they inhibit breathing. Others feel that unless your running pace is relatively slow, frostbite is no problem, even at wind-chill readings of −40 F, and so a mask is not necessary. They claim, on the basis of experience, that running keeps their skin so warm and flushed with blood that frostbite is no danger. Nonetheless, our recommendation is to use a ski mask when wind-chill factors are high. Play it safe.

Another type of mask is designed to filter the polluted air that many people in urban centers have to breathe. If you habitually find yourself jogging alongside cars and trucks spewing out carbon monoxide, a mask of this type might be worth using.

Mittens — Mittens, not gloves, give your hands their best protection in cold weather. Because mittens do not have separate fingers, cold air cannot circulate around each individual finger. With the fingers and the palm of the hand crowded together, nice and warm in the same air space, the heat from each finger mingles with the heat of the other fingers and the palm. Some people use socks as mittens, but in order to keep them from slipping off the hand you generally have to tie something around the wrist. This constriction tends to cut off blood circulation to the hand and is not recommended. Spend a few dollars for a pair of good mittens instead.

Stopwatches

Only advanced runners should use a stopwatch for competitive timing. Anyone else should refrain from turning his or her run-

Other Equipment

ning into a footrace. Don't try to combine time and distance when you run. That is, if you want to run for time, say 30 minutes, then run for 30 minutes without paying much attention to the distance you travel in that time. And if you want to run for distance, don't concern yourself with making it in a certain amount of time. Otherwise you will exhaust yourself. Jack Batten speaks for a lot of exercise experts when he says that, "A stopwatch, just its mere presence, makes a jogger too competitive for his own good. It challenges him and forces him to move beyond the level that suits his rate of progress."

The stopwatch does have one very fine use for either the professional runner or the casual jogger: it can give you a very accurate reading of your heart rate, a requirement of our running program and a good thing to keep your eye on in any distance running. (You can, of course, get a pretty accurate pulse count with the sweep second hand of an ordinary wrist watch as well.)

If you do want to invest in a stopwatch, however, you can expect to spend a fair amount of money. Conventional and digital stopwatches can be worn on the wrist or carried on a cord slung around the neck. Conventional stopwatches, that is, those with hands like a clock, start at about $30. Each is designed for a specific type of timing function. For example, a stopwatch with a 10-second sweep hand will time sprints and short races with great accuracy, clearly showing the time down to tenths of a second. Stopwatches with 30-second and 60-second sweep hands do not record the time with as much accuracy, but they can time much longer races.

Digital stopwatches, however, do not have such limitations. They can time races of any length within reason, depending on the design, and are accurate up to 1/100th of a second. There are many ways to time any running event, each requiring a different function. Some digital watches combine up to four of these functions in the same instrument. The digital versions run about $130. The price of a digital capable of only one of these functions runs about $70.

If you anticipate needing only one function, it is not necessary for you to spend the extra $60 for functions you don't intend to use. On the other hand, if money is no object and you want to play with your stopwatch, the watch people will be more than willing to oblige you.

"Athletic Drinks"

Water serves the body in many ways. Among other duties, it transports electrolytes throughout the body — ions of sodium, potassium, calcium, magnesium, chlorine — which, in turn, go about doing their particular tasks. These tasks are necessary for the continuing health of any body and include the proper functioning of every muscle, including the heart muscle. When you perspire heavily in an extended run, water pours out of you and, with the water, these electrolytes. A chemical balance is created which must be restored.

Several commercial "electrolyte replacement" drinks are currently available for this purpose: Gatorade, Body Punch, QuickKick, to name several of the commonly used brands.

Some veteran runners swear by them, declaring that these fluids helped them break through "the wall" — that moment at about 20 miles when you lose that "spark," your muscles refuse to work, and you just can't go on.

Runners who have had experience with them stress the importance of drinking these electrolyte replacement drinks long before you become thirsty. If you wait until you are thirsty it will be too late.

Despite the enthusiasm of some runners for these electrolyte replacements, the claims made for them have not been established beyond question by any means, and in fact raise a good deal of controversy. In the absence of convincing evidence either way, we do not offer a recommendation. We do stress the importance of nutrition and a diet rich in these electrolytes — leafy greens, grains, fruit, milk, and cheese.

Fun Runs And Marathons

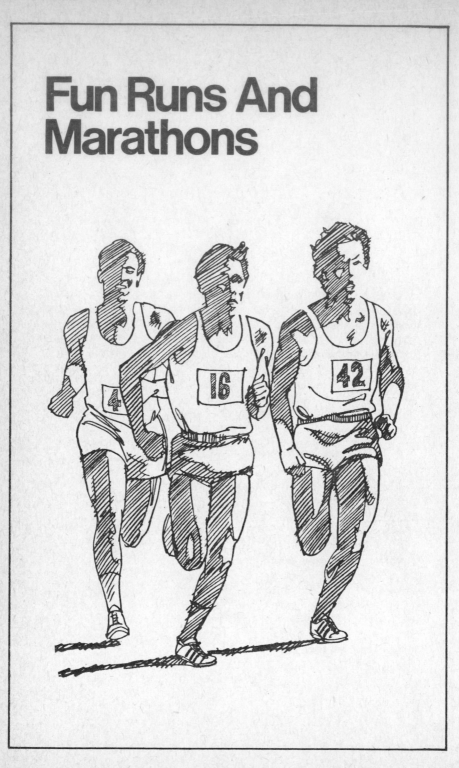

Fun Runs And Marathons

THERE ARE distance *runs* and distant *races*. They may cover the same amount of territory, but the psychological and physical differences between them are substantial.

Distance running is what you do on your own or with a few congenial spirits. Essentially, you are competing with yourself, driving your body on to greater and more satisfying achievements. Your primary concern is improving your own running. In distance racing you compete against the clock, other runners, or both. This requires rigorous training and mental toughness. The potential Olympic champion thrives on competition and is motivated by it to improve his or her own performance. Most of us, though, are not prepared to dedicate our lives to paring down our times. Running is something we do for pleasure and good health, not the major preoccupation of our existence.

These two kinds of events seem poles apart, but a recent development on the running scene is a happy combination of the two.

Fun Runs

Fun runs are organized group runs that are regularly scheduled throughout the year in practically every area of the country as well as in Canada and other foreign nations. The runs, which some consider races and others as workouts or get-togethers, can be as short as a quarter mile or as long as 10 miles.

Fun runs are listed in a directory published by *Runner's World,* which contains location, times, dates, the person to contact, and other relevant information. A complete directory of current fun runs can be obtained free of charge by sending a stamped, self-addressed envelope to:

Fun Run Updates
Runner's World
1400 Stierlin Road
Mountain View, CA 94042

Fun runs are an ideal way to get to know other runners, those who share your interests in the sport. Much valuable information is transmitted from runner to runner — everything from techniques to equipment analysis and the treatment of aches, pains, and other running problems.

Among the greatest advocates of fun runs is publisher-editor Bob Anderson, founder of *Runner's World.* The comprehensive coverage of the events in his publication (updates are included in each issue) have done much to spread their popularity throughout the country. We share his enthusiasm for fun runs and recommend them to runners at all levels. They are appropriately named; they are fun and there are countless other benefits that can come from getting together with other runners.

Distance Races

All track meets feature distance races. Not all of them offer the same ones, nor will one organized meet necessarily have all the major distances. Amateur Athletic Union (AAU) track meets are not that easy to enter; they are usually invitational or restricted in one way or another. There are, however, a lot of other distance competitions that are open to anyone who wants to pay the fee (if there is one) or who has the moxie to sign up.

A great many distance races are now being sponsored by cities and organizations. The recent increase in their number and in the growing roster of participants attests to the growth of running as a sport in America.

This is competition, and it can be strong. Check out the race to be sure it is for people at your level of running competence. It is no fun to run in a race with others who are vastly superior to you.

Marathons

The marathon is the ultimate event for the runner. It is agonizing for body and mind, as brutally demanding as any event or competition in the sports world.

Fun Runs And Marathons

Twenty-six miles, 385 yards is the distance, and the best runners cover it in just a little over two hours. There are no official world records for marathons, however, because, although the distance is standard, the courses vary considerably.

Just think of it. A fast marathoner maintains an average speed of about five minutes a mile for the entire distance of 26 miles, 385 yards. Only a tiny handful of the world's runners can run a single mile in that time, much less 26 consecutive ones. Even a three-hour marathon requires an average of 6.8 minutes a mile, fast by any standards.

Despite the arduous demands of a marathon, thousands upon thousands of runners are competing in hundreds of these races across the country. And sex or age are apparently no deterrents. People over 70 have competed and finished in remarkable times.

The two most famous marathons today are the one held as part of the Olympic Games every four years and the Boston Marathon, which attracts about 5000 runners each year.

How It Began

The race itself commemorates the legendary run of a Greek warrior named Pheidippides in 490 B.C. The Athenians were at war with the Persians, the superpower of the day, and fully expected to be defeated. As the citizens waited for the bad news, the Athenian army won an astonishing victory at Marathon. Pheidippides, after an exhausting day on the battlefield, ran the 26 miles to Athens to inform the people that the danger was over. There is no record of how long this epic run took, but his pace must have been swift, because the legend relates that he fell dead after relaying his message.

Distance races played no part in the Olympics of the ancient world, but they became popular when the Games were revived in 1896, 1500 years after they were abolished by Emperor Theodosius I of Rome. The marathon distance was set at 26 miles. The extra 385 yards were added at the 1908 Olympics in England, the first really successful modern Games, so that the runners could start at Windsor Castle. Since 1908 all marathons have covered this peculiar distance.

World Records For Distance Races

Men's Events

Event	Record Holder	Time	Date	Place
1500 meters	Filbert Bayi, Tanzania	3:32.2	Feb. 2, 1974	Christchurch, New Zealand
1 mile*	John Walker, New Zealand	3:49.4	Aug. 12, 1975	Gothenburg, Sweden
2000 meters	John Walker, New Zealand	4:51.4	June 30, 1976	Oslo, Sweden
3000 meters	Brendan Foster, Great Britain	7:35.2	Aug. 3, 1974	Gateshead, England
3000-meter steeplechase	Anders Garderud, Sweden	8:08.02	July 28, 1976	Montreal, Canada
2 miles*	Brendan Foster, Great Britain	8:13.8	Aug. 27, 1973	London, England
5000 meters	Emiel Puttermans, Belgium	13:13.0	Sept. 20, 1972	Brussels, Belgium
6 miles*	Ron Clarke, Australia	26:47.0	July 14, 1965	Oslo, Norway
10,000 meters	Samson Kimobwa, Kenya	27:30.5	June 30, 1977	Helsinki, Finland
10 miles*	Jos Hermens, The Netherlands	45:57.0	Oct. 13, 1975	Papendal, The Netherlands

* Unofficial record. Distances in miles are not recognized as official world records.

Fun Runs And Marathons

World Records For Distance Races

Event	Record Holder	Time	Date	Place
Men's Events				
20,000 meters	Jos Hermens, The Netherlands	57:31.8	Sept. 28, 1975	Papendal, The Netherlands
25,000 meters	Lekka Paivarinta, Finland	1:14:16.8	May 15, 1975	Oulu, Finland
30,000 meters	James Alder, Great Britain	1:31:39.4	Sept. 5, 1970	London, England
Women's Events †				
1500 meters	Tatiana Kazankina, USSR	3:56.0	June 28, 1976	Podolsk, USSR
1 mile*	Natalia Marachescu, Rumania	4:23.8	May 21, 1977	Bucharest, Rumania
3000 meters	Ludmila Bragina, USSR	8:27.1	Aug. 7, 1976	College Park, Maryland

* Unofficial record. Distances in miles are not recognized as official world records.
† The list is much smaller for women because long distance races for women under official auspices are a recent development. The first Olympic distance race for women (1500 meters) was held in 1972.

Fun Runs And Marathons

Modern Marathons

News of marathons are published in *Runner's World* and in a new magazine *The Marathoner*.

The major annual marathons in the United States and Canada are listed on the following pages. Even if you have no intention of attempting this distance yourself, go down and watch the endurance specialists. They'll appreciate some cheers from the sidelines!

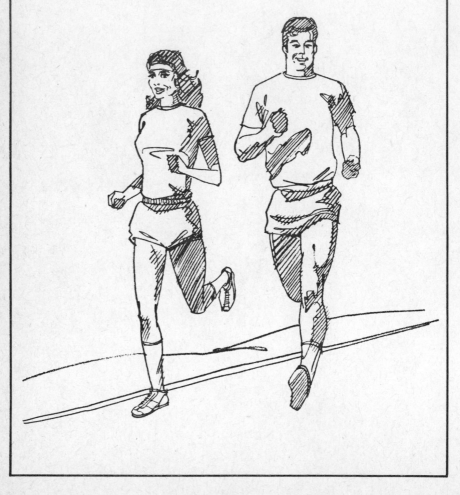

Fun Runs And Marathons

State and City	Marathon	Month Held
Alabama		
Huntsville	Joe Steele Rocket City	December
Alaska		
Anchorage	Mayor's Midnight Sun	June
Eielson AFB	Sun Bear Midnight Run	June
Fairbanks	Equinox	September
Hope	Resurrection Pass	July
Arizona		
Globe	Copper Valley	October
Scottsdale	Fiesta Bowl	December
Tucson	Arizona Admissions Day	February
Arkansas		
Little Rock	Ground Hog Day	January
California		
Bakersfield	Bakersfield	February
Chico	Bidwell Classic	March
Culver City	Western Hemisphere	December
Orange County	Orange County	April
Irvine	Senior Olympics	May
Livermore	Livermore	December

Fun Runs And Marathons

State and City	Marathon	Month Held
Loma Linda	Orange Grove	April
Lompoc	Valley of the Flowers	June
Los Alamitos	Los Alamitos	March
Los Angeles	Los Angeles	March
Madera	Madera	December
Newbury Park	Hidden Valley	February
Orange	World Masters	January
Palos Verdes	Palos Verdes	June
Rohnert Park	Sonoma State	October
Sacramento	Sacramento	October
San Diego	Mission Bay	January
San Francisco	San Francisco	July
San Mateo	West Valley	February
San Pedro	Rose Bowl	November
Santa Barbara	Santa Barbara	October
Saratoga	Paul Masson Champagne	January
Walnut	Mount Sac Relays	April
Weott	Avenue of the Giants	May
Colorado		
Denver	United Bank Mile-Hi	May
Denver	Denver YMCA	October
Dillon	Summit County	August
Manitou Springs	Pikes Peak	August

Fun Runs And Marathons

State and City	Marathon	Month Held
Connecticut		
Middletown	John W. English	March
Florida		
Fort Myers	Florida	March
Gainesville	Florida Relays	March
Melbourne	Space Coast	November
Miami	Orange Bowl	December
Shalimar	Valentine Running Festival	February
Georgia		
Atlanta	Peach Bowl	January
Atlanta	Stone Mountain	February
Atlanta	International Women's Championship-Avon	March
Hawaii		
Hilo	Big Island	July
Honolulu	Honolulu	December
Lihue	Garden Isle	October
Maui	Maui	March
Idaho		
Boise	Les Bois	November
Illinois		
Aurora	Aurora	July

Fun Runs And Marathons

State and City	Marathon	Month Held
Chicago	Mayor Daley	September
DeKalb	DeKalb	April
Flora	CCAP Southern Illinois	September
Hinsdale	Hinsdale	November
Monticello	Freedom	October
Indiana		
Bloomington	Pizza Hut	November
Carmel	Windy	March
Fort Wayne	Three Rivers Festival	July
Terre Haute	Marathon-Marathon	June
Iowa		
Ames	Cyclone Marathon	June
Cedar Falls	University of Northern Iowa	April
Des Moines	Drake Relays	April
Winterset	Covered Bridge	October
Kansas		
Lawrence	Kansas Relays	April
Topeka	Mel Voss Memorial	December
Kentucky		
Lexington	Kentucky Relays	April

Fun Runs And Marathons

State and City	Marathon	Month Held
Louisiana		
Crowley	International Rice Festival	October
Natchitoches	Christmas Festival	December
New Orleans	Mardi Gras	January
Maryland		
Baltimore	Maryland	December
Beltsville	Washington's Birthday	February
Frederick	Life and Health	April
Massachusetts		
Boston	Boston Athletic Association	April
Lowell	VFW	March
Newton	Silver Lake	February
Michigan		
Breckenridge	Breckenridge	July
Detroit	Motor City	October
Port Huron	Oliver "Scotty" Hanton	September
Saginaw	Saginaw Bay	May
West Bloomfield	West Bloomfield	March
Minnesota		
Minneapolis	City of Lakes	October

Fun Runs And Marathons

State and City	Marathon	Month Held
Mississippi		
Clinton	Mississippi	December
Missouri		
Columbia	Heart of America	September
St. Louis	Third Olympiad Memorial	February
Montana		
Helena	Governor's Cup	June
Kalispell	Jerry Anderson	October
Nebraska		
Folk City	Tri-State	October
Omaha	Omaha	August
Nevada		
Incline Village	Lake Tahoe	June
Las Vegas	Las Vegas	February
Reno	Silver State	September
New Hampshire		
Hanover	Dartmouth Medical School	October
New Jersey		
Asbury Park	Jersey Shore	December

Fun Runs And Marathons

State and City	Marathon	Month Held
New Mexico		
Albuquerque	Albuquerque	October
Clovis	Clovis	October
New York		
Albany	Hudson-Mohawk	March
Buffalo	Buffalo to Niagara International	October
Ithaca	Boston Qualifier	March
Ithaca	Finger Lakes	October
Lake Placid	Lake Placid	September
Liverpool	First Trust North Area	May
Plattsburgh	Champlain Valley YMCA	May
Rochester	Rochester	September
Staten Island	New York City	October
Westbury	Earth Day	March
Yonkers	Yonkers	May
North Carolina		
Bethel	North Carolina	January
Charlotte	Charlotte Observer	December
Fort Bragg	All American	November
Greensboro	Greensboro	October
Raleigh	International Masters	May

Fun Runs And Marathons

State and City	Marathon	Month Held
North Dakota		
Grand Forks	North Dakota	June
Ohio		
Athens	Athens	March
Hudson to Cleveland	Revco Western Reserve	May
Monroe	Monroe	October
Toledo	Heartwatchers	March
Toledo	Glass City	June
Oklahoma		
Gage	Roadrunner	May
Tulsa	Oil Capital	March
Oregon		
Eugene	Nike-OTC	September
Portland	Portland	November
Seaside	Trails End	February
Pennsylvania		
Erie	Presque Isle	September
Harrisburg	Harrisburg National	November
Johnstown	Johnstown YMCA	October
North Park	Boston Qualifier	March
Philadelphia	Penn Relays	April

Fun Runs And Marathons

State and City	Marathon	Month Held
Philadelphia	Provident Bulletin	October
Potter County	Gods Country	June
State College	Nittany Valley	February
Trexlertown	Prevention	March
Rhode Island		
Newport	Ocean State	October
South Carolina		
Columbia	Carolina	February
South Dakota		
Brookings	Longest Day	November
Tennessee		
Chattanooga	First Tennessee Bank	November
Oak Ridge	Smoky Mountain	February
Texas		
Austin	Texas Relays	April
Canyon	Palo Duro Canyon	January
Dallas	White Rock	December
Houston	Houston	January
San Antonio	Las Colonias	May

Fun Runs And Marathons

State and City	Marathon	Month Held
Utah		
Promontory to	Golden Spike	May
Brigham City		
Salt Lake City	Desert News	July
St. George	Pioneer	October
Vermont		
South Hero	Green Mountain	August
Virginia		
Richmond	Richmond Newspaper	October
Virginia Beach	Rotary Shamrock	March
Waynesboro	Waynesboro	October
Washington		
Blaine	Birch Bay	April
Cheney	Cheney	November
Seattle	Seattle	November
Spokane	Spokane Heart	September
Washington, DC	Marine Corps Reserve	November
West Virginia		
Huntington	Hall of Fame	March

Fun Runs And Marathons

State and City	Marathon	Month Held
Wisconsin		
Hurley	Paavo Nurmi	August
Madison	Madison	June
Milwaukee	Wisconsin Mayfair	May
New Glarus	Sugar River Trail	October
Wyoming		
Cheyenne	Cheyenne Frontier	March
	Canada	
Alberta		
Calgary	Alberta	May
Manitoba		
Winnipeg	Golden Mile	May
Newfoundland		
St. Johns	Newfoundland	July
Ontario		
Espanola	Northern Lights	June
Ottawa	National Capital	May
Quebec		
Ile D'Orleans	Ile D'Orleans	October
Montreal	Marathon de Montreal	March

Helpful
Sources

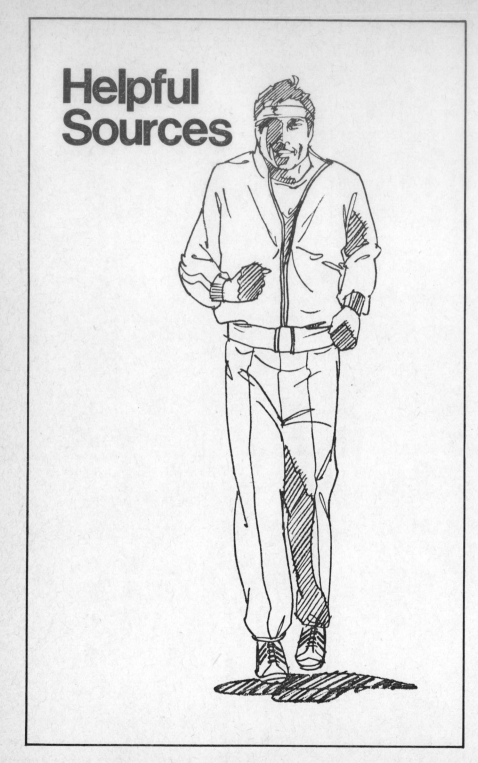

Helpful Sources

DESPITE THE popular myth, the long distance runner doesn't have to be lonely — and neither does the average jogger. All those people you see running down the street are anxious to share their experiences. There are organizations and publications devoted to making that task a little simpler.

The organizations sponsor events, pass on information, and sometimes offer discounts on equipment. At the very least, they provide a sense of community, assuring the runner that a lot of other people are equally interested.

Books on running can be found on library and bookstore shelves across the country. They offer new theories and deeper insights that can enrich your participation and expand your horizons. We have listed the major books on running and some that deal with total exercise programs which emphasize running and cardiovascular fitness.

Magazines and newsletters are the best way to keep up-to-date on what's happening in the world of running. Articles cover a wide range of topics of interest to the runner, including dates and places of events, interviews, advice, and helpful tips. Even the ads can be fascinating reading, keeping you informed about all the latest products.

The American runner is doubly fortunate because there are excellent national and regional publications. The national magazines can usually be found on newsstands. To learn about the regional ones, ask the people at one of the organizations listed. Even easier, ask another runner in your area.

Once you become a runner, you will want to learn more about your favorite sport and meet others who enjoy it too. Take advantage of all these resources. Your running, and your life, will benefit.

Organizations

Especially For Runners

National Jogging Association (NJA)
919 18th Street, N.W.
Washington, DC 20006

Helpful Sources

Road Runners Club of America (RRCA)
1111 Army Navy Drive
Arlington, VA 22202

Other Helpful Groups

American Alliance for Health, Physical Education and
  Recreation
1201 16th Street, N.W.
Washington, DC 20037

American Heart Association
7320 Greenville Avenue
Dallas, TX 75231

President's Council on Physical Fitness and Sports
400 Sixth Street, S.W.
Washington, DC 20201

Young Men's Christian Association (YMCA)
291 Broadway
New York, NY 10007

Young Women's Christian Association (YWCA)
600 Lexington Avenue
New York, NY 10022

The Four
Major Magazines

Runner's World
World Publications
Box 366
Mountain View, CA 94042

This is the front-runner in publications for casual and serious joggers, long distance runners, and competitors. It has been

Helpful Sources

around since 1966 and today it is a first-rate publication with a masthead that reads like a "Who's Who" in running: Joe Henderson, George Sheehan, Joan Ullyot, Hal Higdon, etc. Articles are stimulating and always well-written; a variety of departments offers information on areas ranging from sports medicine and training tips to current events and happenings that the runner should know about.

Occasionally, special issues focus on specific subjects and cover them in depth. The annual issue devoted to rating the running shoes (always October), which we referred to in our chapter on running shoes, is extremely comprehensive, yet clearly helpful to even the newest of runners.

Abundant advertising in the magazine will keep you up-to-date on the latest in shoes, outfits, stopwatches, books, competitions, everything in fact that might stimulate the spending impulse of the runner.

Runner's World is published monthly and is available by subscription or at local newsstands.

The Jogger
National Jogging Association
919 18th Street, N.W.
Washington, DC 20006

This is the official publication of the National Jogging Association, issued 10 times a year. It contains enjoyable and informative articles, and aims to please runners at all levels. It comes automatically with membership in NJA, and that is the only way to subscribe to it. The newsletter is not available on newsstands.

The Marathoner
World Publications
Box 366
Mountain View, CA 94042

The people at *Runner's World* decided the interest in marathoning was growing at such a rapid rate that the subject

Helpful Sources

deserved a magazine all its own. Previously, the topic was covered in *Runner's World*.

The first issue hit the newsstands in April 1978 and this publication seems to be prepared with the same care, imagination, and quality that has always been a part of *Runner's World*.

The magazine is written mainly for the competitive runner, but you certainly do not have to be a marathoner to enjoy and get something out of it. Highly illustrated (including a good amount of color) and attractive in design, it offers thorough in-depth coverage of the marathon scene as well as timely reports on what is going on in the sport.

Published quarterly, *The Marathoner* is available by subscription and at local newsstands.

Today's Jogger
Stories, Layouts & Press Inc.
257 Park Avenue South
New York, NY 10010

This magazine is also a newcomer. Smaller than *Runner's World,* it appears to be aimed at the less experienced runner.

Some impressive names in the field of running have contributed articles (Thaddeus Kostrubala, Charles Kuntzleman, etc.) There is good enjoyable reading here but not a lot of advice or guidance-oriented articles.

Today's Jogger is a bi-monthly publication, offered by subscription and at newsstands.

Books

Ald, Roy: *Jogging, Aerobics and Diet.* New York, Signet (New American Library), 1968.

Anderson, Bob, and Henderson, Joe (eds.): *Guide to Distance Running.* Mountain View, California, World Publications, 1974.

Helpful Sources

Batten, Jack: *The Complete Jogger.* New York, Harcourt Brace Jovanovich, 1977.

Bowerman, William J., and Harris, W.E.: *Jogging.* New York, Grosset & Dunlap, 1967.

Consumer Guide®:*Rating the Exercises.* New York, William Morrow & Company, 1978.

Cooper, Kenneth H.: *The Aerobics Way.* New York, M. Evans & Co., 1977.

Cooper, Kenneth H.: *The New Aerobics.* New York, M. Evans & Co., 1970.

Cooper, Mildred and Kenneth H.: *Aerobics for Women.* Mountain View, California, World Publications, 1972.

Fixx, James: *The Complete Book of Running.* New York, Random House, 1977.

Henderson, Joe: *Joy, Run, Race.* Mountain View, California, World Publications, 1977.

Henderson, Joe: *The Long Run Solution.* Mountain View, California, World Publications, 1976.

Kostrubala, Thaddeus: *The Joy of Running.* Philadelphia, J.B. Lippincott Co., 1976.

Kuntzleman, C.T. (ed.): *The Physical Fitness Encyclopedia.* Emmaus, Pennsylvania, Rodale Books, 1970.

Morehouse, Lawrence E., and Gross, Leonard: *Maximum Performance.* New York, Simon & Schuster, 1977.

Myers, Clayton R.: *The Official YMCA Physical Fitness Book.* New York, Popular Library, 1975.

Helpful Sources

President's Council on Physical Fitness and Sports: Various publications. Washington, DC, Government Printing Office.

Runner's World: *Runner's Training Guide*. Mountain View, California, World Publications, 1973.

Runner's World: *The Complete Runner*. Mountain View, California, World Publications, 1974.

Sheehan, George A.: *Dr. Sheehan on Running*. Mountain View, California, World Publications, 1975.

Subotnick, Steven: *The Running Foot Doctor*. Mountain View, California, World Publications, 1977.

Ullyot, Joan: *Women's Running*. Mountain View, California, World Publications, 1976.

Van Aaken, Ernst: *Van Aaken Method*. Mountain View, California, World Publications, 1976.

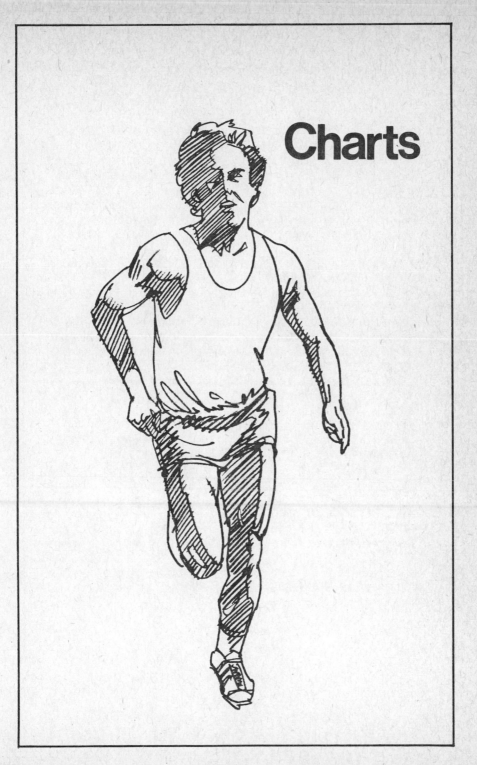

Charts

Reference Charts

ONE OF THE benefits of exercise is weight control. Vigorous physical activity not only burns up calories, but enables you to redistribute your weight and lose extra inches of padding. For these reasons, exercise is an important part of any well-designed diet plan.

The first charts given below are height/weight charts showing ideal weights for men and women of different heights and body types. Height alone is not enough to determine what you should weigh. A person with small bones and a delicate frame, for example, should weigh quite a bit less than a large-boned person of the same height.

Another consideration is the kind of weight your body carries. A heavily muscled athlete or manual laborer can expect to be "overweight" in terms of height and bone structure. As long as this extra weight is muscle rather than fat, it is not a health hazard. On the other hand, a very sedentary individual may be "underweight" but have more fat.

The next two charts show the amount of weight you can expect to lose by regular participation in a running program. These figures are based on additional exercise, excluding any time you have spent on them right along.

The fifth chart is a handy wind-chill factor reference table. Use it whenever you run in cold weather.

Next you will find a summary of the CONSUMER GUIDE® running program. This quick-reference summary contains the basic information you need to follow the program.

The Runner's Checklist is a reminder of the key points to remember during the course of your program. Complying with this checklist will make your running career happier and healthier.

The Runner's Log is designed to help you keep track of your progress. You will be able to see at a glance just how much you have improved.

Reference Charts

Height/Weight Guide For Men

Height*	Small Frame (Pounds)	Medium Frame (Pounds)	Large Frame (Pounds)
6'4 "	164-175	172-190	182-204
6'3 "	160-171	167-185	178-199
6'2 "	156-167	162-180	173-194
6'1 "	152-162	158-175	168-189
6'0 "	148-158	154-170	164-184
5'11"	144-154	150-165	159-179
5'10"	140-150	146-160	155-174
5'9 "	136-145	142-156	151-170
5'8 "	132-141	138-152	147-166
5'7 "	128-137	134-147	142-161
5'6 "	124-133	130-143	138-156
5'5 "	121-129	127-139	135-152
5'4 "	118-126	124-136	132-148
5'3 "	115-123	121-133	129-144
5'2 "	112-120	118-129	126-141

*With shoes with one-inch heels.
Source: Boehringer Ingelheim, Ltd., Elmsford, N.Y. 10523

Reference Charts

Height/Weight Guide For Women

Height*	Small Frame (Pounds)	Medium Frame (Pounds)	Large Frame (Pounds)
6'0 "	138-148	144-159	153-173
5'11"	134-144	140-155	149-168
5'10"	130-140	136-151	145-163
5'9 "	126-135	132-147	141-158
5'8 "	121-131	128-143	137-154
5'7 "	118-127	124-139	133-150
5'6 "	114-123	120-135	129-146
5'5 "	111-119	116-130	125-142
5'4 "	108-116	113-126	121-138
5'3 "	105-113	110-122	118-134
5'2 "	102-110	107-119	115-131
5'1 "	99-107	104-116	112-128
5'0 "	96-104	101-113	109-125
4'11"	94-101	98-110	106-122
4'10"	92-98	96-107	104-119

Note: For women between 18 and 25, subtract one pound for each year under 25.
*With shoes with two-inch heels.
Source: Boehringer Ingelheim, Ltd., Elmsford, N.Y. 10523

Reference Charts

Walking — Exercise/Weight Loss Guide

Minutes Of Walking*	Reduction Of Calories Per Day (In Kcal)	Days To Lose 5 Pounds	Days To Lose 10 Pounds	Days To Lose 15 Pounds	Days To Lose 20 Pounds	Days To Lose 25 Pounds
30	400	27	54	81	108	135
30	600	20	40	60	80	100
30	800	16	32	48	64	80
30	1,000	13	26	39	52	65
45	400	23	46	69	92	115
45	600	18	36	54	72	90
45	800	14	28	42	56	70
45	1,000	12	24	36	48	60
60	400	21	42	63	84	105
60	600	16	32	48	64	80
60	800	13	26	39	52	65
60	1,000	11	22	33	44	55

*Walking briskly (3.5-4.0 mph), calculated at 5.2 Cal/minute.

Source: Frank Konishi, Exercise Equivalents of Foods. (Carbondale and Edwardsville, IL, Southern Illinois University Press, 1974, pp. 21-25, 30-43).

Reference Charts

Running — Exercise/Weight Loss Guide

Minutes Of Running*	Reduction Of Calories Per Day (In Kcal)	Days To Lose 5 Pounds	Days To Lose 10 Pounds	Days To Lose 15 Pounds	Days To Lose 20 Pounds	Days To Lose 25 Pounds
30	400	21	42	63	84	105
30	600	17	34	51	68	85
30	800	14	28	42	56	70
30	1,000	12	24	36	48	60
45	400	18	36	54	72	90
45	600	14	28	42	56	70
45	800	12	24	36	48	60
45	1,000	10	20	30	40	50
60	400	15	30	45	60	75
60	600	12	24	36	48	60
60	800	11	22	33	44	55
60	1,000	9	18	27	36	45

*Running — Alternate jogging and walking, calculated at 10.0 Cal/minute.

Source: Frank Konishi, *Exercise Equivalents of Foods*. (Carbondale and Edwardsville, IL, Southern Illinois University Press, 1974, pp. 21-25, 30-43).

Reference Charts

Wind-Chill Factor Reference Table*

Wind Speed Miles Per Hour	If The Thermometer Actually Reads:											
	50	40	30	20	10	0	−10	−20	−30	−40	−50	−60
5	48	37	28	16	6	−5	−15	−26	−36	−47	−57	−68
10	40	28	16	4	−9	−21	−33	−46	−58	−70	−83	−95
15	36	22	9	−5	−18	−36	−45	−58	−72	−85	−99	−102
20	32	18	4	−10	−25	−39	−53	−67	−82	−96	−110	−124
25	30	16	0	−15	−29	−44	−59	−74	−83	−104	−113	−133
30	28	13	−2	−18	−33	−48	−63	−79	−94	−109	−125	−140
35	27	11	−4	−20	−35	−49	−64	−82	−98	−113	−129	−145
40	26	10	−6	−21	−37	−53	−69	−85	−102	−116	−132	−148

*All temperatures are expressed in degrees Fahrenheit. The wind-chill factor is a combination of actual temperature and wind speed which produces the effect of a lower temperature. For example, a temperature of 50F with a wind speed of 5 miles per hour has the same effect on exposed flesh as a temperature of 48 F.

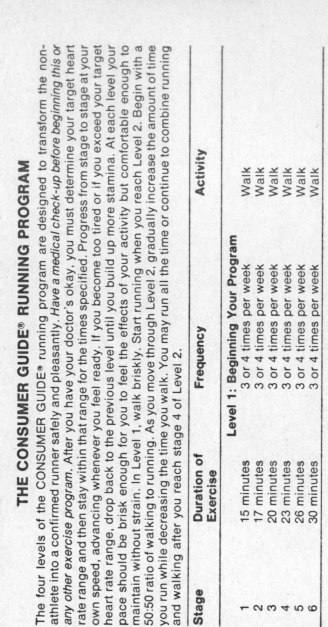

Reference Charts

THE CONSUMER GUIDE® RUNNING PROGRAM

The four levels of the CONSUMER GUIDE® running program are designed to transform the non-athlete into a confirmed runner safely and pleasantly. *Have a medical check-up before beginning this or any other exercise program.* After you have your doctor's okay, you must determine your target heart rate range and then stay within that range for the times specified. Progress from stage to stage at your own speed, advancing whenever you feel ready. If you become too tired or if you exceed your target heart rate range, drop back to the previous level until you build up more stamina. At each level your pace should be brisk enough for you to feel the effects of your activity but comfortable enough to maintain without strain. In Level 1, walk briskly. Start running when you reach Level 2. Begin with a 50:50 ratio of walking to running. As you move through Level 2, gradually increase the amount of time you run while decreasing the time you walk. You may run all the time or continue to combine running and walking after you reach stage 4 of Level 2.

Stage	Duration of Exercise	Frequency	Activity
		Level 1: Beginning Your Program	
1	15 minutes	3 or 4 times per week	Walk
2	17 minutes	3 or 4 times per week	Walk
3	20 minutes	3 or 4 times per week	Walk
4	23 minutes	3 or 4 times per week	Walk
5	26 minutes	3 or 4 times per week	Walk
6	30 minutes	3 or 4 times per week	Walk

206

Reference Charts

Stage	Duration of Exercise	Frequency	Activity
Level 2: Starting To Run			
1	18 minutes	4 times per week	Run/walk/run/walk
2	20 minutes	4 times per week	Run/walk/run/walk
3	23 minutes	4 times per week	Run/walk/run/walk
4	25 minutes	4 times per week	Run or run/walk/run/walk
5	28 minutes	4 times per week	Run or run/walk/run/walk
6	30 minutes	4 times per week	Run or run/walk/run/walk
Level 3: The Accomplished Runner			
1	33 minutes	4 times per week	Run or run/walk/run/walk
2	35 minutes	4 times per week	Run or run/walk/run/walk
3	38 minutes	4 times per week	Run or run/walk/run/walk
4	40 minutes	4 times per week	Run or run/walk/run/walk
5	43 minutes	4 times per week	Run or run/walk/run/walk
6	45 minutes	4 times per week	Run or run/walk/run/walk
Level 4: The Advanced Runner			
1	48 minutes	3 or 4 times per week	Run or run/walk/run/walk
2	50 minutes	3 or 4 times per week	Run or run/walk/run/walk
3	53 minutes	3 or 4 times per week	Run or run/walk/run/walk
4	55 minutes	3 or 4 times per week	Run or run/walk/run/walk
5	58 minutes	3 or 4 times per week	Run or run/walk/run/walk
6	60 minutes	3 or 4 times per week	Run or run/walk/run/walk

Checklist For Runners

This checklist is designed to make your running as pleasant and as safe as possible. Keep it handy and refer to it often.

1. Have a thorough medical examination before you start your program.
2. Set up a graduated series of goals and proceed to accomplish them at your own pace.
3. Warm up before you start your run and cool down afterwards.
4. Include exercises for the rest of your body in your program.
5. Be sure your running shoes fit properly.
6. Wear comfortable clothing that keeps you warm in winter and cool in summer.
7. If you run when it is fairly dark, wear light-colored clothing. Even better, attach reflective strips to your clothes.
8. Run defensively, staying alert for cars, unleashed dogs (and their droppings), holes in the road, and other hazards.
9. Plan your course ahead of time. If possible travel over it before running, checking out the terrain and the conditions.
10. Avoid hard surfaces such as concrete and asphalt as much as possible.
11. Drink plenty of liquids before starting out. Do not drink anything alcoholic.
12. Wait one hour after eating before you run.
13. Always carry a little money with you for emergencies.

The Runner's Log

This Runner's Log is designed to help you keep track of your progress. Remember that the key to a successful running program is maintaining your target heart rate for the specific amount of time recommended for each Level. Under "Type Of Activity" record whether you walked, ran, combined the two in a run/walk pattern, or substituted another cardiovascular exercise such as swimming or basketball.

Runner's Log

Day	Level	Stage	Duration Of Exercise (Minutes)	Type Of Activity
Week 1				
Monday				
Tuesday				
Wednesday				
Thursday				
Friday				
Saturday				
Sunday				

The Runner's Log

Day	Level	Stage	Duration Of Exercise (Minutes)	Type Of Activity

Week 2

Day	Level	Stage	Duration Of Exercise (Minutes)	Type Of Activity
Monday				
Tuesday				
Wednesday				
Thursday				
Friday				
Saturday				
Sunday				

Week 3

Day	Level	Stage	Duration Of Exercise (Minutes)	Type Of Activity
Monday				
Tuesday				
Wednesday				
Thursday				
Friday				
Saturday				
Sunday				

The Runner's Log

Day	Level	Stage	Duration Of Exercise (Minutes)	Type Of Activity

Week 4

Day				
Monday				
Tuesday				
Wednesday				
Thursday				
Friday				
Saturday				
Sunday				

Week 5

Day				
Monday				
Tuesday				
Wednesday				
Thursday				
Friday				
Saturday				
Sunday				

The Runner's Log

Day	Level	Stage	Duration Of Exercise (Minutes)	Type Of Activity

Week 6

Day	Level	Stage	Duration Of Exercise (Minutes)	Type Of Activity
Monday				
Tuesday				
Wednesday				
Thursday				
Friday				
Saturday				
Sunday				

Week 7

Day	Level	Stage	Duration Of Exercise (Minutes)	Type Of Activity
Monday				
Tuesday				
Wednesday				
Thursday				
Friday				
Saturday				
Sunday				

The Runner's Log

Day	Level	Stage	Duration Of Exercise (Minutes)	Type Of Activity

Week 8

Day	Level	Stage	Duration Of Exercise (Minutes)	Type Of Activity
Monday				
Tuesday				
Wednesday				
Thursday				
Friday				
Saturday				
Sunday				

Week 9

Day	Level	Stage	Duration Of Exercise (Minutes)	Type Of Activity
Monday				
Tuesday				
Wednesday				
Thursday				
Friday				
Saturday				
Sunday				

The Runner's Log

Day	Level	Stage	Duration Of Exercise (Minutes)	Type Of Activity
Week 10				
Monday				
Tuesday				
Wednesday				
Thursday				
Friday				
Saturday				
Sunday				
Week 11				
Monday				
Tuesday				
Wednesday				
Thursday				
Friday				
Saturday				
Sunday				

The Runner's Log

Day	Level	Stage	Duration Of Exercise (Minutes)	Type Of Activity

Week 12

Day	Level	Stage	Duration Of Exercise (Minutes)	Type Of Activity
Monday				
Tuesday				
Wednesday				
Thursday				
Friday				
Saturday				
Sunday				

Week 13

Day	Level	Stage	Duration Of Exercise (Minutes)	Type Of Activity
Monday				
Tuesday				
Wednesday				
Thursday				
Friday				
Saturday				
Sunday				

The Runner's Log

Day	Level	Stage	Duration Of Exercise (Minutes)	Type Of Activity

Week 14

Day	Level	Stage	Duration Of Exercise (Minutes)	Type Of Activity
Monday				
Tuesday				
Wednesday				
Thursday				
Friday				
Saturday				
Sunday				

Week 15

Day	Level	Stage	Duration Of Exercise (Minutes)	Type Of Activity
Monday				
Tuesday				
Wednesday				
Thursday				
Friday				
Saturday				
Sunday				

The Runner's Log

Day	Level	Stage	Duration Of Exercise (Minutes)	Type Of Activity

Week 16

Day				
Monday				
Tuesday				
Wednesday				
Thursday				
Friday				
Saturday				
Sunday				

Week 17

Day				
Monday				
Tuesday				
Wednesday				
Thursday				
Friday				
Saturday				
Sunday				

Index

Index

Index

Index

M

N

O

P

Index